Women and Health:
Tradition and Culture in Rural India

MRIDULA BANDYOPADHYAY
Hong Kong University of Science and Technology

STEWART MacPHERSON
City University of Hong Kong

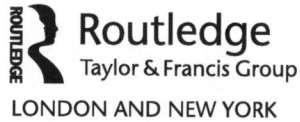

Routledge
Taylor & Francis Group

LONDON AND NEW YORK

First published 1998 by Ashgate Publishing

Reissued 2018 by Routledge
2 Park Square, Milton Park, Abingdon, Oxon, OX14 4RN
52 Vanderbilt Avenue, New York, NY 10017

Routledge is an imprint of the Taylor & Francis Group, an informa business

Publisher's Note
The publisher has gone to great lengths to ensure the quality of this reprint but points out that some imperfections in the original copies may be apparent.

Disclaimer
The publisher has made every effort to trace copyright holders and welcomes correspondence from those they have been unable to contact.

A Library of Congress record exists under LC control number: 97077384

ISBN 13: 978-1-138-35878-2 (hbk)
ISBN 13: 978-1-138-35882-9 (pbk)
ISBN 13: 978-0-429-43412-9 (ebk)

WOMEN AND HEALTH: TRADITION AND CULTURE IN RURAL INDIA

Contents

List of Tables and Figures

Preface

The present study explores the health situation of 402 ever married women in four districts of West Bengal state, India, and is based on empirical data. A survey was conducted in late 1993 and early 1994 to collect data on maternal and child health in rural India. The main focus of the study is on socio-economic and cultural factors influencing maternal and child health care practices, health care behaviour, reproductive health, family planning, perception about illness and disease, and utilisation of health care resources.

The main findings suggest that with increasing socio-economic status of the family, and development of the village, health care behaviour of the people changes drastically. More women accept family planning and small family norm, irrespective of religious beliefs or caste, and are more likely to utilise the available health care resources. However, the study reveals that irrespective of socio-economic status, religion or development, age at marriage remains very low, suggesting the influence of cultural pressures to marry early and to have children immediately. Son preference is found to be very strong. Postnatal care is found to be minimal because of lack of awareness and knowledge regarding postnatal services and its benefits and also because of the belief that it is not essential and necessary.

Medical pluralism is prevalent; more than one medical system is used simultaneously, depending on the perceived severity of illness. Treatment is sought from any or all of the available medical facilities (traditional, homeopathy, ayurvedic, or allopathic). A further finding indicates 'consumer oriented' health care behaviour for perceived major ailments and 'welfare oriented' behaviour for perceived minor ailments. Depending on the perceived severity of illness the study population oscillate between either 'consumer oriented' or 'welfare oriented' health care behaviour and utilisation.

Since the study was conceptualised with exploratory, descriptive methodology and framework in mind, advanced levels of quantitative analysis were not thought to be an appropriate tool to explore the social and cultural aspects influencing maternal and child health. Given the characteristics of the data, the study describes in detail with the help of frequency tables the relationship and association between different variables. However, tests of significance were performed to see the relationship between various socio-economic variables and health care behaviour and utilisation. The tests have not been included in this book, if anyone is interested to know more about the tests and results, please contact the authors for more information.

Finally, I would like to thank my friends and colleagues in India; Prof. U. P. Sinha, Prof. Tara Kanitkar, Prof. T. K. Roy, Mr. Deshpande, Dr. B. M. Ramesh, and Dr. A. G. Khan from the International Institute of Population Sciences (IIPS), Bombay, India, who helped and supported me immensely during the course of my field work, and data analysis. Prof. Paul Wilding and Prof. Veronica Pearson contributed substantially to this study with their creative suggestions and criticisms. I would also like to thank my colleagues and friends in the Department of Public and Social Administration, City University of Hong Kong. Lastly, I would like to thank Dr. Joe Thomas, my partner, for all his support and help and surviving my flare-ups and encouraging me through out the entire process of writing this book.

Mridula Bandyopadhyay

List of Abbreviations

ANM	Auxiliary Nurse Midwife
AWW	Anganwadi Workers
BEE	Block Extension Educator
BPHC	Block Primary Health Centre
CHC	Community Health Centre
CSSM	Child Survival and Safe Motherhood
DMO	District Medical Officer
IAS	Indian Administrative Service
ICDS	Integrated Child Development Services
LHV	Lady Health Visitor
MCH	Maternal and Child Health
NHP	National Health Policy
PHC	Primary Health Centre
PHN	Public Health Nurse
TBA	Traditional Birth Attendant
UN	United Nations
VHG	Village Health Guide/Volunteer Health Guide
WHO	World Health Organisation

Introduction

Despite the rising living standards and modern health care in the developing countries, a wide gulf exists between the have and the have-nots. The poor and rural women, urban slum dwellers, squatters, and indigenous population are primarily at the receiving end of the inequitable growth in most of the developing countries of the world. India is no exception to this kind of existential and urban oriented development. Because of marginal development, often the poor and the women are the most affected. The health status of a population is a reflection of the socio-economic development of a country and is also an indicator of social well-being. It is important to have a healthy population for progress and development. In the words of Subedi,

> The health of a population is an important element in its ability to progress and develop. If health is to be improved in a population - particularly in developing countries - health services must be capable of delivering effective health care and members of the population must use these services (Subedi, 1989, p. 412).

Health and health care utilisation in developing countries reveal significant disparities between women and men. Women in the developing countries often suffer from poor health, but consume less health care resources than males. Women in the developing countries are also often confronted with numerous socio-cultural factors which negatively encroach upon their physical well-being and access to appropriate health care services. Even though female children start out with a genetic advantage, socio-cultural factors intervene and the biological advantage is wiped out by the end of their lifetime. Though men and women have similar health needs, a woman also has additional health needs and problems, primarily related to her reproductive and nurturing roles. For a woman in a developing country, the childbearing years are the most risky, due to factors including poor communication and transportation, lack of adequate pipe-borne water and generally low standards of living (Ojanuga and Gilbert 1992; Sundari, 1992; Stinson, 1986; Momsen, 1987; Rutter, 1988; Stock, 1983; WHO, 1985).

Nearly 500,000 women die every year from complications of childbirth or pregnancy related problems. Difficulties that some women experience during labour are directly attributable to nutritional stunting as a result of deficient diets. The laborious work that women are required to perform, has a detrimental effect upon their health and, in certain circumstances, upon the viability of their babies. Nearly one-third of the infants die each year in the developing countries due to infectious diseases and diarrhoeal infections (WHO, 1992, 1986; Karkal 1985; Acsadi, and Johnson-Acsadi, 1991; UNFPA, 1988; UNICEF, 1984).

Though efforts have been made to make health care available to all the people by the national governments of every country in the world, the most deprived people are the poor rural villagers and urban slum and squatter settlement dwellers. Moreover, women in general are the marginalised population deprived of modern health care, especially reproductive health, in many countries of the developing world (WHO, 1992).

Principle Theme

Many factors affect women's reproductive health care behaviour and children's health in rural India. Even though innumerable factors augment women's reproductive health care behaviour and children's health in rural India, only a limited number of issues related to utilisation of health care both for women and children have been looked into.

Often, complex interaction between a host of factors and women's health contribute to morbidity and mortality of infants and mothers, low birth weight babies, health problems after delivery, and sometimes complications during pregnancy, labour and delivery. There are also many other important issues such as economic decision making regarding health care utilisation, preference and expenditure on a particular illness, etc. are also part of the universe under study. The scope of this book however, is limited to the following areas. How socio-economic and cultural factors contribute towards shaping the health of women in general and how the socio-economic and cultural factors affect health and nutritional status of the mother, reproductive status, utilisation of health services, awareness of health services, health care behaviour, cultural practices associated with child birth, lactation, and so on.

What is Health

The World Health Organisation (WHO) and the United Nations Children's

Fund (UNICEF) organised the Alma-Ata Conference in 1978 on Primary Health Care, which prepared the ground for national government efforts to establish community-based primary health care programmes in many developing countries. As stated in the Declaration of the 1978 Alma-Ata Conference on Primary Health Care, health is defined as:

> a state of complete physical, mental and social well-being and not merely the absence of disease or infirmity, it is a fundamental human right and ... the attainment of the highest possible level of health is a most important world-wide social goal ... (WHO, 1978).

The right to the enjoyment of good health as a basic human right has also been affirmed by the two United Nations Symposia on Population and Human Rights (UN, 1974, 1981). The Alma-Ata Conference in 1978 was an important milestone in the struggle for health. The conference was organised in response to the widespread dissatisfaction with existing health services in the late 1960s and early 1970s. Despite the efforts by different countries and the World Health Organisation (WHO) to improve and extend health services, large numbers of people, particularly in the rural areas of developing countries, were left with no access to health care. Hence, primary health care was seen as the route to health for all. Since the formulation of the goal of 'Health For All By The Year 2000,' countries throughout the world have made efforts to strengthen and expand their systems of primary health care.

Health For All by the Year 2000 AD, has been accepted by most nations as a worthwhile goal. The central theme of Health For All, is 'universal access to health care.' If attained, 'Health For All by the Year 2000,' would ensure all people of the world a level of health that would make it possible for each individual to lead a socially and economically productive life (Mahler, 1981).

Despite all these goals and targets set up by various international organisations, 'Health For All' has not yet been fully realised by many developing nations, as evidenced by the continued under development of health and health care resources in many developing areas of the world.

What does Health Mean to People in India

Health involves the interplay of socio-economic and cultural factors. Health as a concept varies from culture to culture. The concept of health and disease are all shaped and fashioned by culture. Due to the cultural differences different communities perceive health and disease differently and accordingly health care behaviour varies depending upon the norms, values, beliefs, social taboos, food avoidance, and socio-cultural practices, and so on (Park and Park, 1991). Indians, be it Hindus, Muslims, or any other group of people belonging to different castes and communities, recognise illness as either due to external agents, such as injuries, poisons and possession by evil spirits, or due to intrinsic upsets of physiological regulators caused by an unhealthy life style or an incorrect dietary intake. Illness is explained by sins in this or past lives and salvation lies in acceptance of suffering. Religious activities are the first, and often only, reaction to illness (Ghadiali, 1983).

Due to the cultural and geographical differences and variations, the perception of health and practices of health care behaviour varies. The concept of personal hygiene and community and societal hygiene too varies according to the culture and environmental conditions. Clearly, geography, cultural area, and the relative position of women are important as a woman's health is a good indicator of the status of women in a society. As such, to explain these variations it is necessary to study a society from the different angles influencing health.

All people strive for a long and healthy life; and the provision of such a life is a goal of all societies. Hence, the role of health care is crucial in any development process. Therefore, the emphasis on health care should shift from disease and disability cure to the care aspect and recognise the importance of all aspects of the health system—preventive, promotive, curative and rehabilitative.

Health Situation of Women and Children in India

As health is an important component of social well being, different countries in the world have different health policies as regards to their environment, geographical location, etc. India, too has its own health policies which were implemented after its independence. The Government of India has initiated a number of programmes to control and eradicate communicable and epidemic diseases and to prevent health hazards to improve upon the nutritional status of the people and in general to raise the standard of health of the people. In order to achieve this numerous Primary Health Care Centres (PHC) were made available in the rural areas of India (WHO, 1992; Sinha 1990).

Various development programmes have been launched by the government to improve the standards of living to achieve a stable and healthy population. That women often receive inadequate health care is increasingly being recognised. On the whole women are exposed to the same illnesses as men, although they have special health needs: they are likely to carry a heavier workload than men, and to spend many years in pregnancy and lactation. Despite these difficulties, the low status of women in many societies often results in their receiving an inadequate diet—putting further strain on their health—and having less access to health care. In response to the inequality and discrimination faced by women, the United Nations proclaimed 1975-85 to be the Decade for Women. This created a new awareness of the problems, but the effects have yet to be felt in the lives of most women (WHO, 1992; Smyke, 1991).

Though a large number of studies exist on women and health in the developing countries (Vlassoff, 1994; Okojie, 1994; Maine, 1987; Basu, 1990; Sundari, 1992; Key, 1987; Smyke,1991; Kielmann, 1983; Khan, 1988; Visaria, 1985; Ojanuga and Gilbert, 1992), there seems to be a lack of studies done in India on the utilisation of available health care services, health care behaviour, and factors inhibiting utilisation of the available modern health care, especially during the reproductive phase of a woman's life.

Methodology

An anthropological approach was used in data collection. Along with in-depth interviews, and non participant observation, a survey was conducted on maternal and child health care in four selected villages of West Bengal state, with emphasis on women's reproductive health, family planning, children's health care, and utilisation of health care resources for adults and children. In addition, in-depth case studies on cultural practices related with pregnancy, labour, delivery and postpartum period were also collected from women respondents. As the study was conceptualised with exploratory, descriptive methodology and framework in mind, advanced levels of quantitative analysis were not thought to be an appropriate tool to explore the social and cultural aspects influencing maternal and child health care. The data collected was mainly nominal in nature. Given the characteristics of the data, the present study describes in detail with the help of frequency tables the relationship and association between different variables.

Selection of the districts and villages

Data was collected from four different districts representing different levels of socio-economic development, access to health care institutions, status of women, communication, transportation, and religion. Interviews were conducted with 400+ women in the reproductive age group of 13-49 years. A detailed interview schedule was prepared to collect data on socio-economic aspects, housing conditions, and health care issues. The questionnaire contained 184 questions, both structured and open-ended, and took almost an hour and a half to two hours to complete. In addition, in-depth case studies on practices related with pregnancy, labour, delivery and postpartum period were also collected from women respondents.

To make a representation of the whole state, the districts and villages were chosen in such a manner so as to assimilate the diverse cultural, religious, and socio-economic heterogeneity of the state. There are 17 districts in the state of West Bengal. Out of these 17 districts, four districts were chosen to make a representation on the basis of socio-economic development, access to health care institutions, status of women, communication, religion, etc. Accessibility to these areas was also taken into consideration.

One village from each district was chosen on the basis of socio-economic development, religion, status of women, etc. The developed area chosen was socio-economically advanced as compared to the other study districts, in terms of the overall economic condition of the district, communication, accessibility, transportation, heterogeneity of the population and education. Whereas the underdeveloped area was chosen on the basis of 'Birth Rate' exceeding 39.5 (definition of an underdeveloped area according to the Indian Census).

The study was undertaken in the districts of Puruliya, Medinipur, Murshidabad and Barddhaman in late 1993. All the districts and villages had a Primary Health Centre (PHC) located within a vicinity of five kilometres or so.

Village Motipur, District Puruliya (Under-developed area)
The total population of the village of Motipur according to the 1981 census (1991, village level statistics are not yet available) is 1318 out of which 406 persons are literate (31%). The village is almost entirely inhabited by tribals and scheduled castes (68%), and there are a total of 228 households in this village.

Village Kapgari, District Medinipur (Hindu Area)
This village was predominantly inhabited by Hindus, barring a few households. According to the 1981 census (1991, village level statistics are not yet available), the total population of the village is 1368 out of which 809 persons are literate (59%), and there are a total number of 212 households in the village.

Village Santoshpur, District Murshidabad (Muslim Area)
This is the only district in the state of West Bengal with a majority and high concentration of Muslim population. The total population of the village is 876 out of which 88 persons are literate (10%). The village is almost entirely inhabited by Muslims, and there are a total of 152 households in this village.

Village Sultanpur, District Barddhaman (Developed and Heterogeneous Area)
According to the 1981 census (the village level data of the 1991 census is not yet available), the total population of the village is 1562 out of which 670 persons are literate (43%). The village is inhabited by people belonging to different caste and tribal groups and also to different religious groups and sects. The village has scheduled castes, scheduled tribe population, and also people from the Hindu and Muslim faiths. There are a total of 270 households within the village.

Selection/identification of households in the villages

One hundred households were selected randomly from each village. The random selection of the households were based on a voter's registration list which was obtained from the 'Gram Panchayat Office'. Every other household was picked randomly and identified from the voter's list for the sole purpose of survey. An official from the Panchayat Office escorted the research team to each household which was picked from the voter's list and introduced the research team to the head of the households and to the family members, and explained the purpose of our visit, and requested their full co-operation.

Selection of informants/respondents

From each household, one woman respondent was selected on the basis of her marital status, age, and parity. Only one woman from each household was chosen, because if there were more than one eligible women in the household, it was presumed that they would all have similar belief patterns, practices, taboos, and similar behaviour towards health and health care utilisation. The women respondents were selected in such a manner so as to make a representation of all the age groups between 15-45 years.

About a third of the women from each age group were selected (13-24; 25-34; 35-49). Besides, the women were also selected on the number of children they had and on their current marital status. This kind of sampling was employed to observe the differences and similarities in health care utilisation of women and their family members, family planning practices, utilisation of health care for children, use of antenatal, postnatal and other available reproductive health services, and also to find their opinion about the existing health care facilities, perception regarding different illnesses, and so on, between the different generations of women in the sample.

Besides, individual case studies were also conducted with the help of in-depth interview schedules. Cultural practices related to pregnancy, childbirth and lactation vary within each caste, tribe and religion, hence case-studies were conducted within each type of caste, tribe and religious groups. Influence of traditional health care was looked into and the influence of ethno-medicine (Shamanism) was also explored. Field observation schedules were developed to generate additional data on health care behaviour, related to sanitation, hygiene, environmental factors, utilisation of health centres and traditional health care systems.

The entire process of data collection from four villages, of 100 households each, took roughly about four months. Four research assistants were appointed to help with the data collection. Before going to the field the research assistants were trained in conducting person to person interviews, and all the other factors associated with the data collection. All the four research assistants and the researcher tried to be present at each village for the interviews. The total number of respondents were 402 women in the age-group of 13-49 years. The interviews were conducted in Bengali.

Problems Faced in the Field

Co-ordinating a team of four research assistants and making travel, food, lodging and boarding arrangements was a huge problem, as there were constant complaints by the research team on the inadequacies of the living quarters, plumbing, water and electricity, mode of transportation, quality of the food, and so on. Apart from these inconveniences, other problems related to the data collection were also encountered in the field.

Person-to-person interview sessions turned into a free for all discussion and it was very difficult to get the respondent alone with the interviewer. Then there was the time and availability factor, when the women were free at a stretch for two hours to answer all the questions. Recall lapses (about births, deaths, stillbirths, exact dates of events, age, etc.) were encountered frequently as a majority of the respondents are illiterate and did not remember dates, and times, or birth-weights, etc.

The tribal women were hostile and suspicious and refused to answer any questions. It took a lot of convincing and frequent visits to their homes to obtain the relevant information. Most of the time the standard reply for most questions was "Don't Know" or "God's wish/punishment", it took a lot of probing and prodding to elicit replies to certain questions.

Normally the respondents and their relatives wanted to know the purpose of the whole exercise and asked if they would benefit in some way if they spent two hours of their time answering all our questions.

Presentation of Chapters

This book is divided into nine chapters. Chapter two discusses certain critical issues related to maternal and child health and focuses on the socio-cultural factors affecting health of women and children. It further outlines an analytical framework for examining maternal health in rural India.

Chapter three presents an overview of the study area and profiles the study area and its population with regards its geographical location, physical setting, demographic characteristics, socio-economic conditions of the households surveyed and also the health care perception, behaviour, and utilisation, of the population. It further reviews the health situation of India and state of West Bengal. This section details the mortality and fertility situation in the country and major states.

The focal point of chapter four is the social context of women's health in rural India. Chapter five summarises and outlines the attitude towards utilisation of available health care services and family planning needs and its effect on women's health.

Chapter six primarily concentrates on the utilisation of health care services during pregnancy, labour and delivery, and after childbirth; that is, utilisation of antenatal, and postnatal services, and utilisation of health care services during labour and delivery. Chapter seven summarises the cultural practices followed after childbirth, especially abstinence and food taboo during lactation. Chapter eight discusses the health status of infants and children under five years of age, with special reference to their weight at birth, breast feeding and weaning practices. Further it details the utilisation of health care services and immunisation for infants and children. Chapter nine presents an overview and summarises the major issues.

Maternal and Child Health: Certain Critical Issues

Extensive literature is available in the area of maternal mortality, morbidity, and health. However, often the focus is on the issues related to status of women, under-development, poverty, reproduction related mortality, socio-cultural factors affecting health of women, indices of women's' health status such as life expectancy, access to health care, gender discrimination and family planning.

There are very few studies of the various cultural factors affecting women's health in rural India. Though nearly 500,000 women die each year as a result of pregnancy and childbirth in the developing world, and maternal mortality in India is one of the highest in the world, ranging from 500-800 per 100,000 births (WHO, 1986; Karkal, 1985), most of the studies and researches concentrate on the directly responsible obstetric causes of death, or access to health care services. Very few authors have studied the underlying cultural and traditional practices and factors related to pregnancy, childbirth and lactation. Most of the available literature is on maternal mortality and child survival, and most are of a descriptive nature or quantitative studies. Hence, there is a need to develop theoretical models for explaining the inter-relationships between various factors associated with maternal health in rural India, as very few studies have tried to explain the entire process or pathways through which maternal health is affected. Therefore, an attempt has been made to present a detailed conceptual framework to analyse maternal health in rural India.

Factors Affecting Women's Health

Indices of Women's Health Status

Life expectancy of a population is one of the most useful measures in assessing health status of a given society and its population's well-being. Normally, the female foetus has a higher survival rate than the male foetus. In addition women usually live longer than men, in most countries (Stinson, 1986; Momsen, 1987).

11

Hence, it would seem that women should have a significantly higher life expectancy than males. Yet in many developing countries, a wide gap exists between male and female life expectancy. In India, Nepal, Bangladesh, and parts of the Middle East, life expectancy for males has been significantly higher than females (Stinson, 1986; Momsen, 1987; Rutter, 1988). Moreover, the mortality rates for female children are usually higher than males during the early childhood years (1-4 years) in India, Nepal, and Bangladesh (Sinha, 1990; Jain, 1985; Visaria, 1988).

Female babies have a certain built-in genetic advantage over boys, and ordinarily one would expect to find about 117 male infant deaths to every 100 female. But, according to Ravindran (1986),

In countries where the social status of women is very low, the lack of care received by girls and women is so great that this environmental disadvantage far outweighs their genetic advantage ... This may result in a complete reversal of the usual trend of higher male infant and/or child mortality in these countries, and a greater proportion of female infants and children die here than male. Excess female infant and child mortality may therefore be seen as a warning signal indicating the serious neglect of girls in the society concerned (Ravindran, 1986, p. 12). It is estimated that 'every sixth death of a female infant in India, Bangladesh and Pakistan is due to neglect and discrimination.' In India alone this would amount to over 300,000 girls per year (Ravindran, 1986, p. 12).

The widely used indicator for judging the general well-being of women is life expectancy. Life expectancy tells us little about the quality of health during life. In three countries of South Asia (India, Nepal and Pakistan) the difference in life expectancy is in men's favour and the years in which this reverse differential is most common are early childhood and the childbearing years (Key, 1987, p. 59).

The frequency of higher female mortality in both Asia and Africa during childhood years is associated with the relatively low cultural position accorded to girls and women. In the rural areas of Asia and Africa, a boy is much more highly valued than a girl for his economic potential and is given correspondingly greater care (Ojanuga and Gilbert, 1992). In India, for example, 23 per cent of girls and only 19 per cent of boys die before the age of five years (Momsen, 1987).

Life expectancy for women in India is lower than it is for men. This lower female life expectancy is due to higher female mortality up to 35 years of age with particularly large differentials in the 0-4 and 15-29 year age groups. In some parts of India, especially the northern states, the female infant mortality rate is considerably higher than the males and female deaths are said to occur because of neglect of female children (Chatterjee, 1985).

In societies such as India, higher mortality for females is a reflection of the role and status of females, both within the family and in society at large, as much as they represent the health consequences of social, economic and cultural discrimination against them (Karkal, 1987, p. 1343).

In developing countries the health of women plays a very important role in determining the overall mortality levels. The majority of the population in the developing countries suffer from a number of communicable and non-communicable diseases, and lives in environmental conditions that are hazardous to health. Men and women have similar health needs, but women also have their special health needs and problems, primarily related to their reproductive and nurturing roles (WHO, 1985).

Status of Women

The status of women in a society is a significant reflection of the level of social justice in that society, and involves a complex set of interrelated factors. Women's status is often described in terms of her level of income, employment, education, health and fertility, as well as the role she plays within the family, the community and society. It also involves society's perception of these roles and the value it places upon them. What women do (their work in agriculture or industry, their contribution to the family income, household maintenance, community organisation and development, and their role in the family and the bearing and rearing of children) not only affects their health but is also affected by it (WHO, 1985).

The high level of mortality seen in the developing countries is but one dimension of the problem of poverty; other dimensions are low levels of literacy and low productivity because of poor health, lack of skills and inability to acquire physical capital (World Development Report, 1980). Poverty has a direct impact on women's health besides the status of women in the family, community and society. Women are the bearers and rearers of children; they are responsible for caring for the household; they are often food producers and almost always food processors and servers; they are fetchers of water and fuel; they are the ones who care for the sick and elderly, they are breadwinners as part of the paid labour force, as traders, or by selling items produced at home; they are very often the volunteers working on community projects; in some societies they must be hostesses, chauffeurs, and so on; they are in reality the transmitters of cultural and religious traditions, although seldom are they the authority or official spokesman in this realm (Smyke, 1991).

Under Development

> The consequence of under-development often affect the most vulnerable members of the community at a disproportionate rate. Gender specific analysis of health and health care utilisation in developing countries reveal significant disparities between women and men. Women in the developing countries often suffer from poor health, but consume less health care resources than males. In addition to the usual threats to health, such as infectious diseases, poor sanitation, and inadequate water supplies, women in the Third World countries are often confronted with numerous socio-cultural factors which negatively impinge upon their physical well-being and accessibility to appropriate health care services (Ojanuga and Gilbert 1992, p. 613).

Mortality has been found significantly higher among rural than among urban residents in developing countries. For example, in India, infant mortality has been found to be significantly higher among rural (98) than among urban areas (58). Likewise, overall mortality too has been found to be higher in the rural areas (11.1) than in the urban areas (7.1). The excess of rural over urban mortality is partly attributable to the differential distribution of socio-economic characteristics in urban and rural areas. Better educated and higher income people live in greater proportion in cities, as health manpower and facilities are concentrated in the cities (WHO, 1976; Sample Registration Bulletin, 1989).

Large mortality variations among geographical locations such as districts and provinces as well as considerable differentials by ethnicity and religion have been found in some developing countries, particularly in Africa (Farah and Preston, 1982). This trend has also been found in India, for example, Dyson and Moore (1983, p. 42) found that 'in contrast to the north, states in the south and the east are characterised by ... lower infant and child mortality'. The authors attributed these regional differences to lower autonomy of women in the northern kinship system and suggested that 'even ... in the absence of modern health education and services-differences in kinship structure and female autonomy between north and south may influence patterns of child care, and hence child mortality' (p. 50). On the other hand, Nag (1983, p. 895), attributed the lower mortality in Kerala 'mostly to its higher social development and partly to its favourable environmental and hygienic conditions'.

However, the death rate in rural areas is uniformly higher than that in urban areas in all the states and union territories, except in Kerala, Daman and Diu. The death rate in the age-group (0-4) is the single most important factor causing wide variations in the death rates. Mortality in the early ages is uniformly high in rural areas in all the major states, except Kerala (Sinha, 1990). Official estimates of the prevailing mortality situation of the country reveal that children below the age of five, specially in rural areas, are the worst sufferers (Sample Registration Bulletin, 1988).

Reproduction Related Mortality

In most developing countries, women of reproductive age (15 to 49 years) constitute a little more than one-fifth of the total population. These women are exposed repeatedly to the risk of pregnancy and childbearing and, under the existing socio-economic conditions and inadequacies of medical and health facilities, are at a great risk of morbidity and mortality from causes related to pregnancy and childbirth (Bhatia, 1993).

In India as in other South Asian developing countries and regions, pregnancy and childbearing have from time immemorial impaired women's health and shortened their lives. The bearing of children in India, remains the most important contributor to adult female mortality. For a woman in a developing nation, the childbearing years are the most risky as every year about 500,000 women die of complications of pregnancy, and childbirth, most of them preventable. 'In the developing countries, reproduction related mortality is universally the first five leading causes of death for women in the 15-45 year age group' (Howard, 1987).

Generally, the main causes of maternal deaths are haemorrhage, often with anaemia as an underlying cause and, sepsis (WHO, 1985). Over half of the world's maternal deaths occur in South Asia, predominantly in Bangladesh, India and Pakistan. In South Asia each year, 300,000 women die—and many more suffer from serious illness or permanent disability due to pregnancy-related causes. The region accounts for 27 per cent of the world's births, but more than one half of all maternal deaths (Safe Motherhood Conference, 1990).

The maternal mortality rate in India is estimated to be around 40 per

10,000 births, with a range from as low as 10 per 10,000 births in Kerala State to over 100 per 10,000 births in Madhya Pradesh and Rajasthan (Rao, 1985). Most statistics on maternal mortality are based on hospital and health centre records and thus exclude very many women from rural areas. Therefore, the estimates of maternal mortality in India vary considerably. Estimates based on civil registration systems at the national level were 460 maternal deaths in 1984 and 340 in 1985 per 100,000 live births (Rao, 1985; WHO, 1986).

However, most estimates of MMR in India are based on fragmentary information based on only a small segment of the population. The hospital statistics upon which many estimates are based are not drawn from representative samples of the total population, since an overwhelming majority of deliveries in India, as in many other developing countries, are conducted by traditional birth attendants (TBAs) (Bhatia 1982a; 1982b; and 1985).

Many abortions are performed in rural areas of India by unqualified medical practitioners, and numerous women have continued to use TBAs even after the enactment of the Medical Termination of Pregnancy Act (1971), which liberalised the practice of induced abortion (Bhatia and Mehta, 1972; Bhatia, 1973). A large proportion of these abortion-related deaths are not included in maternal mortality estimates. However, abortion related deaths constitute a major proportion of maternal mortality in India (Rao and Malika, 1977).

Even though a registration system for vital statistics is well established in India, births and deaths are severely under-registered, and the rates obtained directly from civil registration data do not provide adequate information for estimating the level of maternal mortality. Available evidence is incomplete with regard to population coverage, medical certification of the causes of deaths, and classification procedures. As a result, reported maternal deaths constitute only a fraction of the total deaths (Puffer and Griffin, 1967).

In a developing country like India, the socio-economic, socio-cultural and general health factors affecting maternal mortality are much more important than the directly responsible obstetric or medical causes. Besides the socio-cultural and economic factors, there are a number of reasons why women in the rural areas of India do not seek medical care during pregnancy and delivery (Sundari, 1992). The staggering toll that reproduction takes upon women in India, and in some other developing countries, is caused by old-fashioned traditions, social customs, harmful marital and reproductive patterns. Many diseases, health impairments and deaths related to reproduction are preventable and can be warded off by following sound norms and practices relative to marriage, childbearing and the condition and status of women in the family and society (Acsadi and Johnson-Acsadi, 1991).

Other health care behaviours are also likely to have important influences on the outcome of pregnancy for women. Though abortion is legal in India, many women are unaware of this fact and use the services of illegal abortionists to terminate an unwanted pregnancy. Abortions, both induced and spontaneous, are widespread in the developing countries. Induced abortion is probably the most widely used method of limiting the number of children or terminating an unwanted pregnancy. WHO estimates that illegal abortions kill up to 200,000 women a year and permanently injure the health of countless more. Moreover, harmful but traditional practices during pregnancy and childbirth like decreasing the quantity and quality of food intake or observing food taboos, delivering at home assisted by friends and relatives and cutting of the cord with non-sterilized instruments also contribute to a high maternal mortality rate in most of the developing countries.

> The argument has been advanced persuasively that maternal mortality reflects more than the hazard of a single birth, that it is not a chance event, but one that is more often the culmination of a life of protracted malefic experiences (Royston and Armstrong, 1989).

In addition to the medical complications, bio-social factors equally contributes towards maternal mortality in the Third World countries (Ojo and Savage, 1979). Lack of adequate pipe-borne water and generally low standards of living are the contributing factors in high maternal mortality rates in many of the developing nations (Ojanuga and Gilbert, 1992).

Access and Utilisation of Health Services

Poor communication and transportation systems prevent women from delivering in the hospital. Improving the spatial accessibility of health care is an important issue in developing countries because of mobility limitations. Motorised transportation is still a luxury in many developing countries. Many patients have to walk and few have access to motorised transport. As a result utilisation falls rapidly with distance from a facility (Stock, 1983).

Health care services are increasingly seen as a major proximate determinant of decreased mortality in a population. But it also seems that the mere provision of services does not lead to their better utilisation. In a statewide analysis of infant mortality in India, Jain (1985) concluded that the effective variable of female literacy affected infant mortality mainly through its association with the use of medical facilities. Therefore education of women greatly changes the traditional balance of familial relationships with profound effects on child care with increasing use of the medical facilities (Caldwell and McDonald 1982).

Utilisation of health services is positively influenced by factors such as female literacy, political awareness, and so forth. Nations states that 'the success of health interventions rests on an ability to conform to people's lifestyles' (1985). Cultural or regional identity has an important bearing on the knowledge, attitudes, and practices relevant to the use of health care facilities. Deep cultural beliefs and practices also exist that obstruct advances in socio-economic factors such as education, and that affect regional differences in the position of women (Basu, 1990). For example, traditional marriage and kinship patterns lead to a very different kinds and levels of female autonomy and freedom in the northern and southern parts of the country (Dyson and Moore, 1983).

The situation of women in relation to the health care system, and how they access it is dependent on variables such as their status in a specific culture and society to which they belong, that is, questions related to gender and control of decision-making, their socio-economic situation, the degree of social investment in women, their position in the labour force, and in some instances their ethnicity (MacCormack, 1988; Schultz, 1989). Distance from a health facility is a substantial barrier in receiving medical care. In addition cultural mores dictate that women should not travel unaccompanied. Hence a trip to the hospital may represent a substantial consumption of limited resources in terms of money and work time lost for adult male relatives who must accompany the women and children to the health centre (Booth, and Verma, 1992). It has been found in Punjab that the rate of hospital admissions for girls is lower than for boys and is congruent with social factors that result in a strong son preference. The presence of a dowry system, a culture in which sons inherit land and are responsible for taking care of elderly parents, and the lesser socio-economic worth of women, who are less educated and less likely to work outside the home than men all results in and contributes towards a strong preference for sons (Booth and Verma, 1992; Miller, 1981).

Access to obstetrical care in rural areas constitutes a major determinant in the health outcome of the mother and child, accounting for more complicated deliveries, higher rates of premature babies, as well as increased costs of neonatal care. Most of the health care takes place in the home which is for the most part the responsibility of women who take care of children and relatives (Chavkin and St. Clain, 1990). Women of lower socio-economic status and rural women in developing countries suffer disproportionately from complications of pregnancy and childbirth. They are exposed to greater health risks associated with the lack of safe drinking water, since they usually carry water, wash in rivers or other contaminated sources, cook, and are therefore more exposed to infections than men (Feijoo, and Jelin 1989).

Differential access to health care technologies is also common in developing countries. Some health technologies in the developing countries have been intrinsically inequitable and benefit only a small minority of urban, affluent women. Poor and rural women often have no access and no knowledge about modern health care resources (Cassen, 1982). Availability of services proximate to where people live may influence the magnitude and bulk of visits, more than the rate of utilisation. Hence, mere provision of services does not necessarily lead to their utilisation if the rural women are ignorant or resistant to the services provided by the health centres.

It has been suggested that access to health care services is itself insufficient (Bitran, 1988). Bitran advocates consumer involvement. Under this assumption, in addition to being able to use services, people must also be able to make demands on the system, for better service. Nag (1983) noted from his study on 'Impact of Social and Economic Development on Mortality: A Comparative Study of Kerala and West Bengal,' that the mere existence of health services was not enough. He found that in spite of greater economic development in West Bengal, the mortality levels were much higher compared to Kerala, which had a lower mortality rate. He attributes this to Kerala's politically aware population which made sure that the state's health facilities were evenly distributed; and the highly literate female population has been more disposed to use the health facilities once they became accessible.

A study among Nepali women demonstrated an inverse relationship between contraceptive use and travel time to a facility (Tuladhar, 1987). Lack of adequate clinic facilities in many developing areas of the world, as well as social deterrents to visiting a publicly visible clinic are important determinants of whether women in developing countries utilise the available facilities.

The structural barriers to health care, such as doctor/patient ratio, spatial accessibility, technological interventions, and other factors also affect the utilisation. However, in most of the developing countries, women may further be subjected to institutionalised discrimination in the service delivery system.

Socio Cultural Factors

The major socio-cultural factors which are responsible for the high levels of maternal and child mortality are the status of women in the family and society; as it affects every facet of a woman's life and is a powerful determinant of their health and their children's health. The second factor is the traditional customs concerning marriage which include acceptance of an early marriageable age and encouragement of pregnancies at an early age. Cultural demand for children, especially sons constitute the third factor which contribute towards high levels of maternal, infant and child mortality in the developing countries of the world (Acsadi, and Johnson-Acsadi, 1991). Besides these factors, several other customs and traditional practices are harmful for the health of mothers and their children.

According to a WHO study births to women who are not fully mature can permanently injure their health, and the maternal mortality rate in this age-group is often three times higher than that in the 20-24 year age-group. Whereas, at the other extreme, when children are born to women over 35 years of age there is a higher risk of infant and maternal mortality and morbidity, including congenital malformations. Repeated childbearing, short birth intervals and pregnancy at an early age all pose high risks to the health of women. The significance of women's reproductive and nurturing roles for health and development as a whole is undeniable. The biological and social realities of their maternal role are closely linked to their health status and are major factors in the problems they face in health, employment, education, and many other areas (WHO, 1985).

Preference for Home Delivery

The high maternal mortality rates in most of the developing countries despite advances in health care is mainly due to the attitude of the people, perceptions regarding health and health care, illness, and utilisation of health services, cultural beliefs, taboos, social norms, practices and values, which seem to be of vital importance in accelerating maternal morbidity and mortality. Besides the socio-cultural and economic factors, there may be a number of reasons why women do not seek medical care during pregnancy and delivery. The first of these may be due to a lack of awareness of the seriousness of the problem and the common belief that childbearing is a normal process and nothing could go wrong with such a natural process. For instance, in a progressive state like Maharashtra, the rural women do not use the available maternal and child health (MCH) facilities as they do not feel any need for such services because their parents had safe childbirth without any MCH care provided by the public health system (Mukhopadhyay, 1987).

Moreover, in most of the developing societies, the hospitals or health centres are traditionally associated with sickness and death, where the woman would be attended to by strangers, in the absence of her family and friends. Besides, pregnancy and childbirth are considered to be a natural process and a pleasant experience for women. Hence, women on such occasions prefer to be surrounded by relatives and friends. Moreover, the possibility of being attended by male doctors is unacceptable in some cultures, and the non-tolerance by hospital staff of cultural practices related to childbirth, and the total lack of sympathy and understanding on the part of health personnel discourages women from wanting to deliver in any health centre. Lastly, a large number of rural women believe that childbirth does not need any medical interference and hence prefer giving birth at home surrounded by relatives and friends (Sundari, 1992).

In some areas of India, traditional practices during pregnancy and childbirth include deliveries at home assisted by either female relatives or traditional birth attendants, generally known as *dais* who have little knowledge of modern concepts of health and hygiene. In most of the cases of deliveries at homes assisted by *dais*, kitchen knives, scissors or blades are used to cut the umbilical cord. The outer tip is burnt and a turmeric and castor-oil paste is applied (within India different regions have different practices). These instruments are normally not sterilized and fully boiled water is seldom used (the practice is to use warm water). The risk of early childhood and maternal infections, especially tetanus, is therefore great (Shariff, 1987). Despite the unnecessary suffering and deaths caused by lack of appropriate care during pregnancy and childbirth, only about 60 per cent of births in the world are assisted by trained attendants (WHO, 1985).

Child Birth as 'Natural Event'

It is a common belief in the rural and poorer sector of Indian society that pregnancy and childbirth are natural events of life and no medical treatment or supervision is necessary. The concept of regular antenatal check-ups has not yet developed. This is not only because of low literacy and lack of awareness/knowledge regarding the importance of utilisation of antenatal, natal and post-natal check-ups, but also because of the fact that there are no health care centres in many villages.

For services to be effective, women have to use them. The use of prenatal care (to diagnose either pre-existing health problems or to detect certain complications) and the use of care during and after labour and delivery (to treat complications that may arise then) are particularly important in the case of maternal mortality (McCarthy and Maine, 1992, p. 27).

Son Preference

Almost all societies have valued sons more than daughters ... Even when there is no preference for sons, very few cultures actively prefer daughters. Son preference can mean that a female child is disadvantaged from its birth. It may determine the quality of parental care and extent of investment in the child's development. In extreme cases, son preference may lead to abandonment of female infants or even female infanticide, but its most common form is sheer neglect of girls. Son preference is both a consequence and a cause of the low status of women. It is a consequence because it arises as a result of women being considered as playing only unimportant roles and thus being valued less; and a cause, because this undervaluation in turn leads to lower investment in females and as a result of which they are only able to play a peripheral role in society - causing a further lowering of their status. In either case, it indicates the pervasive prevalence of sexism, where allocation of prestige, power and resources depend on the physical characteristic of sex (Ravindran, 1986, p. 2).

Where son preference is a factor, women continue childbearing until they have sons. This cultural factor causes women to continue childbearing at too advanced an age, when the hazard of mortality is especially great for both the mother and the infant. Childbearing is commonplace among women who are either too young or who are beyond safe childbearing age. They nonetheless attempt to have children, especially sons is an indication of the contribution that they are expected to make to the family and society (Acsadi and Johnson-Acsadi, 1991).

Within India, there is a great diversity as regards culture, tradition, religion, tribal and ethnic groups, as well as the system of law and government. However, one cultural factor that is common to all relates to the value of children and family. Children are a source of prestige, and sons give the family dignity and status, including economic and political power, and ensure that the lineage is perpetuated. Though girls are not welcome in most Indian societies (with a few exceptions), they are an asset in terms of caring for their siblings, help with the housework and farming, cooking, fetching water, and fetching firewood from far away places.

The reasons for son preference vary with the cultures and customs of different societies. In some religions a son is needed to carry out ceremonies for deceased parents. Where the family name is preserved only through male descendants that can be one reason for the preference. Boys may be seen to have a greater economic value if their labour is required on the farm, if only males can own or inherit land, or if they are expected to support elderly parents. Girls, on the other hand, may be looked upon as an additional expense with little return, especially in societies where the tradition of dowry is strong and where a wife goes to live with her husband's family. In some societies boys are highly valued as potential soldiers, heroes, protectors of family and society. Rituals, folk sayings and proverbs reflect the lesser value given to girls (Smyke, 1991, p. 30). A Telugu saying reflects the preference of sons over daughters in most parts of India, 'Raising a girl is like watering a plant in your neighbour's garden.'

A study based on interviews with widows in India found that the value of sons was not so much economic as cultural for the women. Having been conditioned to the values of their society, they found self-fulfillment in having sons. It gave them status in the community (Vlassoff, 1988). Therefore, women want to have sons because their status is enhanced in the community and society. Barrenness subjects a woman being shunned, and her husband might marry again because of the importance of children, especially sons, for achievement of respect, status, power and old age security. Because of this fact, women knowingly shoulder multitudinous risks to their health and life in order to have many children, especially sons.

Moreover, having no other means of adequately caring for herself in later years or attaining some status in society, she will eventually have to depend on her children for economic and moral support (WHO, 1985). Society determines how status is to be defined and, in societies, women achieve recognition and status through childbearing. In as much as this is their ultimate function, and because nature has provided for it, little is invested in their growth and development (Acsadi and Johnson-Acsadi, 1991). The situation is exacerbated by a preference for sons, a tendency that can be seen in many countries and, in its extreme form, is exemplified by abandonment of female infants. The milder manifestation of this is increased fertility and reduced spacing between births and sex differentials in feeding patterns and other socio-economic factors (WHO, 1985). Whatever the root causes for son preference, wherever it is pronounced the resulting discrimination against daughters begins very early in life and is normally accompanied by discrimination in the feeding and care of infant females and even older girls.

Demand for Children

High levels of infant and early childhood mortality and demand for two or more male offspring are the most common reason for the demand for children. The main channel through which these societies influence replacement, is through a fertility regulatory system. The system of social norms, values, customs, laws and institutions relating to family and kinship, sexual relationships, marriage, children, fertility and related matters, embodies many important aspects of life. It is an inseparable part of culture, a part that is strengthened by particular religious beliefs, ideology and/or morality. Its elements are sanctioned by tradition, customary or codified law, and are enforceable by the kinship circle, community or a larger social group. Early and universal marriage and mating, condemnation of childlessness and reluctance to accept contraceptive practices before completing the desired family size, support the demand for a number of children, especially sons (Acsadi and Johnson-Acsadi, 1991).

On an average, rural women in India spend about 16-20 years of their lives carrying and bearing children. The low prevalence of contraceptive use and the denial of personal responsibility for conception (i.e., the widespread notion that God gives children) contributes towards the demand for a number of children. Although these customs and notions are slowly changing, they are still widely prevalent and play an important role in conditions of maternal and child health, and mortality.

Sex Discrimination in Food and in Health Care

Though every stage in a woman's life cycle is filled with health hazards in the developing countries, women tend to utilise health facilities less than men and women themselves tend to favour males over females. This tendency of favouring males over females continues throughout a woman's life cycle, thus aggravating the problem of discrimination against them (Ojanuga and Gilbert, 1992).

Poor and under-nutrition is one of the major and leading cause of low status of women's health in developing countries. Half of African women, two thirds of Asian women, and one sixth of Latin American women suffer from nutritional anaemia, as a result of insufficient quantities of nutritious food (Rutter, 1988). The gender specific analysis of food allocation, distribution and consumption reveals a wide dissimilarity between the sexes. This discrimination in health care and food is a reflection of the role and status of women, both within the family and society at large, which represent the health consequences of social, economic and cultural discrimination against them. Nutritional deficiencies in females stem, at least in part, from the inequitable distribution of food among boys and girls, male and females. Poor nutrition for females does not necessarily begin in the child bearing years, but commences almost from their birth; with differential treatment regarding food intake - boys are given a preference over girls. The boys and men of the family are fed first, and the remaining/leftover food is for the women and girls (WHO, 1985; Acsadi and Johnson-Acsadi, 1991; Basu, 1989, 1989b; Chen, Huq, and D'Souza, 1981). Adult women are also the victims of discriminatory practices in food allocation, as there is a custom in India and the entire sub-continent for the women to eat after the men and children have eaten what they want. Thus the women tend to get the left-over food which is normally insufficient and is of poorer nutritional quality.

Some cultural restrictions related to food habits may be selectively imposed on infants and children, some on women, particularly on widows, pregnant women and women in the initial stages of lactation. In fact food taboos and prejudices are intimately interwoven with the cultural and religious beliefs of each social group. In some cultures customs restrict women from eating foods which are high in protein and certain foods which are protein rich, which are only eaten by men. The daily diet of rural women is seldom nutritionally adequate; it becomes less so during pregnancy and lactation due to various cultural taboos and restrictions.

This discrimination in food distribution between the sexes since childhood, affects the growth of girls and hence results in a short adult height and small pelvis. Due to insufficient nutrition, the small pelvis becomes a major risk hazard to the health of women and results in both obstructed labour, and babies with low birth weight and lessened viability. Underweight infants are particularly susceptible to infections and death during the first year of life (United Nations, 1986).

> Certain difficulties that some women experience during labour are directly attributable to nutritional stunting as a result of diets deficient in protein, calcium and vitamin D. These nutritional deficiencies in females stem, at least in part, from the inequitable distribution of food among boys and girls, male and females (Acsadi, and Johnson-Acsadi, 1991, p. 77).

This type of gender bias may be indicative of the under-evaluation and subordination of females, which is culturally ingrained in some regions of the developing world. Such discrimination can have adverse health consequences for women that may be severe during pregnancy, delivery and lactation (United Nations, 1986). Ruzicka and Chowdhury (1978) observed that in Bangladesh, Pakistan and in parts of India, the disadvantage of girls begins during the post neonatal period. Gopalan (1985, p. 162) supports this observation and says that 'the relative neglect of the female child is evident from the fact of greater prevalence of growth retardation even in infancy among girls than in boys. It is such nutritional 'insult' commencing right from infancy and continued through all stages of development that eventually results in poor maternal health/nutritional status which harms not just the women but the succeeding generation as well.'

> In India, a clear regional pattern of sex differentials in childhood mortality is observed with girls in the northern and northwestern parts of the country faring much worse relatively to boys than in the south. Differential use of health care by the two sexes is probably an important factor. Difference in the amount and kind of medical care provided during illness is also an important determinant of the differences between the sexes (Basu, 1989, p. 194).

A review of the health problems of women in India claims that, like the rest of the developing world, most morbidity and mortality is made up of nutritional and childbirth - related illness (Chatterjee, 1985). Food intake of pregnant women, far from being increased in accordance with need, is further restricted in quantity by religious taboos and fear of a prolonged labour. Children are breastfed for at least two years, yet food intake during lactation does not improve (Rao, 1979). Maternal nutritional depletion is a serious problem for Indian women. Consequently the rate of anaemia among rural and poor urban women is very high.

Some of the cultural beliefs and practices also put women in a disadvantageous position and aggravate the problem of malnutrition among them. For example, it is a commonly held belief that the process of delivering a large child is very painful and could prove risky for both mother and child, and therefore, that pregnant women should avoid high calorie diets (Khan, 1988). Similarly there is a belief in some sections of the population that pregnant women should not eat more food, as it will make the baby big and cause problems to the mother at the time of childbirth. Hence, an undernourished mother faces increased risk from pregnancy and is likely to give birth to an underweight or even stillborn child. Similar dietary restrictions deprive post-partum and lactating women of some of the more nutritious ingredients at a time when they are particularly needed. The quality and quantity of breast milk is also adversely affected by such a diet.

Khan (1987) has gathered evidence indicating discrimination against daughters in the duration of breast feeding, other feeding and medical care in India. The mothers internalise the cultural norms in their infancy and early age. It leads them to give priority to their sons and husbands over their daughters and themselves, in every respect. In some developing countries, where son preference is predominant, there are differential feeding patterns for male and female children. For example, in Punjab, male infants are breast fed longer and given greater quantities of food after weaning than are females. Similar practice of providing larger quantities of food for male children is also found in Matlab, Bangladesh, where boys are given more food than girls after weaning resulting in higher mortality and morbidity rates for females (MacCormack, 1988; Miller, 1981).

In a study in an unspecified region of South Asia, Gopalan and Naidu found that while the incidence of kwashiorkor syndrome (protein deficiency) was 33 per cent higher among girls than boys, 13 per cent more boys than girls were admitted to the hospital for treatment (Gopalan, and Naidu, 1972). Similarly, Chen et al., observed in Bangladesh that 66 per cent more boys than girls under the age of five years were brought in for treatment, although no gender differences in general morbidity were found (Chen, Huq, and D'Souza, 1981). In times of food shortage the nutritional needs of males are given a higher priority than females. This preferential treatment often leads to higher age specific death rates for females under five years of age (Ojanuga, 1991).

Apart from discrimination in food distribution, poverty may also be responsible for the lower intake of protein and other necessary vitamins. However, lower protein consumption and protein malnutrition problems are related to diet pattern and food culture in most parts of India. General poverty has often been exaggerated in explaining the nutritional deficiencies in diets and related diseases in India. Most dietary diseases are related to rigid food preferences, taboos, apathy and/or ignorance (Myrdal, 1968).

According to Myrdal (1968), the causes of malnutrition are popular preferences for foods with little or no nutritional value, irrational food habits, some of which are sanctioned by religion. The taboos, prejudices, irrational beliefs and attitudes centering around food are cultural practices that act as blocks preventing full utilisation of the available food and thus aggravating the state of malnutrition. Diet variations are wide in India and offer a large variety of diet preferences which vary with age, sex, religion, caste and economic status in the same areas, but also vary from place to place producing distinct regional dietary patterns based on availability of food stuff, religious beliefs, customary inhibition and even personal prejudice.

Malnutrition, including anaemia, is a serious health problem, especially in women who have too many pregnancies too closely spaced. The woman's nutritional status, in turn, influences her chances of having a normal delivery and a child with an adequate birth weight as well as her ability to breast-feed without hampering her own health. Nutritional anaemia is widespread among women of child-bearing age and contributes significantly to maternal morbidity and mortality in developing countries (WHO, 1985). WHO estimates that nearly two-thirds of pregnant and one-half of non-pregnant women in the developing countries are affected with anaemia. The high prevalence of anaemia among women is particularly serious in view of their heavy workloads.

High female death rates from medical conditions such as gastroenteritis, colitis, (broncho) pneumonia, tuberculosis, avitaminosis and other diseases associated with malnutrition are frequently indicative of the late stage at which treatment is sought for females (Momsen and Townsend, 1987). This type of gender discrimination reflects the cultural biases of devaluation and subordination of women often found in patrilineal ideology. Moreover, India's health programmes include a large share of health budgets devoted to major hospitals in urban centres and a consequent relative neglect of the rural health infrastructure and a medical profession whose orientation is towards high technology, curative medicine and urban style of life (Cassen, 1982).

Work Load

> The contribution of women to the family and to the economy has not been evaluated, quantified or even recognised. For women grow most of the developing world's food, market most of its crops, fetch most of its water, collect most of its fuel, feed most of its animals, weed most of its fields. And when their work outside the home is done, they light the third world's fire, cook its meals, clean its compounds, wash its clothes, shop for its needs, and look after its old and its ill (WHO, 1992, p. 22).

Women do almost all the world's domestic work; provide more health care than all organised health services put together; grow half the world's food, but own only one per cent of the world's land; make up one-third of the world's paid labour force, but are concentrated in the lowest paid occupations; earn less than three-quarters of the wages of men who do similar work

(Cancellier 1986). Women are half the world's population, but receive one-tenth of the world's income, account for two-thirds of the world's working hours, and own only one-hundredth of the world's property (ILO, 1980).

In addition to the unequal distribution of food, the laborious work that women routinely perform, too, has a detrimental effect upon their health and, in certain circumstances, upon the viability of their babies. The deleterious effect of hard labour for many hours daily, is exacerbated by the nutritional deficiencies from which many of the women suffer, especially during pregnancy and lactation. Furthermore, many women spend hours daily, carrying firewood and water that their families require. In addition, they care for the children, the sick, the older family members, prepare the food, and also care for the home. From about age seven, daughters work alongside their mothers, whereas sons are not required to do so (UNFPA, 1988). In the developing/under-developed societies these tasks are considered to be the duties of women, even during advanced stages of pregnancy. Due to this, women give birth to low birth-weight babies, one of the more sensitive indicators of the probability of infant and early childhood survival and development (Fathalla, et al., 1989).

In rural Uttar Pradesh, women have to do strenuous work even during their pregnancies. Labour intensive family activities, coupled with general poverty, hardly allow them to take any rest or proper food (because of differential food distribution and consumption). Their food intake is far below the minimum calorie requirement of a normal adult woman. Thus, low calorie intake and high consumption of calories due to strenuous physical labour create severe malnutrition and abnormally low haemoglobin levels among pregnant mothers. This leads to various complications, including premature labour, high perinatal mortality and delivery of low birth weight babies (Khan et al., 1987).

Studies clearly show that women engaged in heavy labour during pregnancy have a mean pregnancy weight gain several kilograms less than other women who have a similar food intake. The birth weights of their babies are similarly lower, thus diminishing the babies' chances of survival and healthy growth and development (WHO, 1985).

Consequences of Early Marriage and Childbearing

Age at first marriage and childbearing is an important factor as it affects women's health. Although the age of marriage and first pregnancy is rising in many developing countries, there are still many countries in which over 50 per cent of the first births are to women aged less than 19 years (WHO, 1985). Age at marriage, age at birth of first child, birth order, family size and length of inter-birth interval all have important effects on both infant and maternal mortality and morbidity (Hobcraft 1985; Dyson and Crook 1984; Acsadi and Johnson-Acsadi 1986). Mothers under 18 years of age run a high risk of complications and/or death in pregnancy and childbirth and of giving birth to premature babies. These deaths can be prevented by the postponement of marriage until physical maturity is reached and by better access to family planning services (Key, 1987).

Early marriage is the rule in most of the Indian societies though the legal age of marriage is 18 years for women. But, the weight of tradition guaranteeing protection of the purity of the bride is enough to defy the law. A study of women's age at marriage in Orissa demonstrates an encouraging increase in recent years (Kanitkar and Sinha 1985).

Early marriages and sexual unions are associated with premature childbearing that often leads to infertility, several other ailments or even maternal death. They not only affect the timing of the reproductive process and the lifetime fertility of women, but also, have a marked and unfavourable impact on the viability of offspring. The risk of dying before reaching the end of first year of life is higher for infants born to mothers who are closer to the lower (15-19 years of age) and upper (34-49 years of age) limits of the reproductive period than to those who are in their prime of their child bearing ages (20-29 years of age).

It is a very common practice in rural India for women to be married before reaching the age of 15, at the onset of the reproductive life-span, and to be exposed to pregnancy risks soon after marriage, while still very young, to the extent that they may be physiologically immature for mating and childbearing. In most parts of rural North India, the parents marry off their children when they are little, as young as five years, and when the girl attains puberty she is sent to her in-laws/husband's place for consummation of the marriage. This increases the risk of pregnancy at a very early age (sometimes as early as 13-14 years of age), resulting in high maternal mortality and invariably high infant mortality as well. In the rural areas almost all 17 and 18–year–old–women are married and have at least one to two children. However, hardly any of the married women in these age groups use contraceptives (Mishra, 1984).

Marriage in India, and the sub-continent, is universal. In India, where the age at first marriage is low, the potential for large families is extremely high, with the average number of births being greater than in societies where marriage occurs at a later age. In addition, the proportion of women never married remains very low, because of the universality of marriage. In traditional societies like India, it is a somewhat difficult question to answer as to who decides regarding the reproductive behaviour of a couple. Most of the marriages are normally arranged and the ages at marriage for most of the women are well below the legal age. Usually women tend to marry unknown persons, out of their kinship circle and lineage line and normally into another village. Almost universally a woman has to take up residence with her husband's family. In such societies, there is little room for individual decision-making regarding how many children a couple want to have, at what intervals, when to cease childbearing, or whether to use contraception or not. The proper ways are prescribed by the cultural norms, customs and relevant behavioural patterns, and are sanctioned by the society and tradition (Dyson and Moore, 1983).

In such marriages, there is hardly any communication between the husband and the wife. The communication channel is either linked through the mother-in-law or any other elderly female relative residing in the household (in the absence of mother-in-law). The mother-in-law decides about the reproductive behaviour of the couple, and all the other aspects of the couples life. In such an arrangement the delivery of one child is evidence that the marriage is sound and infertility is grounds for sending the bride back to her own home. The new bride/daughter-in-law in an Indian family is accorded her rightful status only after she produces a child - more often than not only after she produces a male child (Dyson and Moore, 1983).

Dyson and Moore (1983), illustrate how cultural differences between the north and the south of India bear on the age of marriage, fertility, mortality, and fertility regulation. Differences in kinship relations between the north and south of India have critical implications for interspouse communication, female autonomy, and decisions on fertility. Women in the north marry at an earlier age and are subjected to strong pronatalist pressures. According to Dyson and Moore (1983), 'A married woman's prime task is to produce male heirs for the descent group, and, other things being equal, this sex preference in itself will tend to engender higher fertility'.

Caldwell et al. (1982), in their study of an area in Karnataka state, India, paid close attention to the forces of cultural change relating to fertility decisions, including relations between young couples and parents. These relations differ from region to region in India. They also found that Muslims were only half as likely as Hindus to practice family planning and showed significantly higher fertility. Regional differences in attitudes toward family planning are present in most countries, and tie into religion, ethnicity, and similar influences. Even when individuals state that they would like fewer children or accept family planning methods to make that happen, they may take no direct steps to limit fertility or may stop such actions if they face even minor problems. Cultural definitions affect not only the strength and direction of attitudes toward fertility control, but norms on how seriously one should pursue related actions. In a community there can be tightly structured social relations, including hierarchies of occupations, that preclude changes in the traditionally expected numbers of children.

The majority of females in India have little autonomy, are provided with little education and are married at an early age. Their economic activity and freedom of movement are restricted, and they have little input in important decisions affecting their families. The major restraint on the practice of family planning by women is related to their status and stems from a number of social factors and attitudes. Women do not exhibit high risk behaviours of their own choice, but are conditioned to accept and display them by their social environment. The conditioning begins in early childhood, persists throughout their lives and is passed on to their female offspring (Acsadi and Johnson-Acsadi, 1991).

Education Differential and Maternal Education Levels

The level of literacy among adult females in India and other developing countries of South Asia is considerably lower than among adult males. Education bias is most pronounced in South Asia, the Middle East, North Africa, and parts of sub-Saharan Africa, but exists to some extent in almost every region in the developing world (Curtin, 1982). More recently, however, the number of girls enrolled, reached or at least approached, the number of boys. However, at higher levels of schooling, the discrepancy between the sexes still exists.

Generally, female illiteracy is more prevalent in the Asian countries, and particularly in the Islamic countries. More than four women in five in Pakistan (87%), Bangladesh (71%), and Nepal (92%) cannot read. In Nepal, 95 per cent of women have no formal education. The disparity between the educational levels of men and women is particularly pronounced in some of the developing countries, such as Jordan and Turkey, where about half of all married women are illiterate compared to only 13 per cent of their husbands. The common element among countries in which less than 11 per cent of the female population is literate is poverty (Momsen and Townsend, 1987).

In India, although all the state governments, and the central government have made school attendance of both girls and boys compulsory, secondary school attendance is still relatively low for girls in most of the rural areas except for Kerala and a few other states. 'Refusal to educate girls (at least on a par with boys) serves deliberately to cement women's "place" in the society, to solidify their roles and to assure conformity with traditional norms' (Acsadi and Johnson-Acsadi, 1991, p. 77; Belsey and Royston, 1987). Thus, as girls enter puberty, they face a variety of life-threatening health hazards, that, owing to poor health and lack of education, they are inadequately equipped to withstand.

> Lack of education among older women also contributes to the widespread self-neglect characteristic of many women. Such women tend to be inattentive to their own illness and health needs and fail to seek care. It is for lack of education and its corollary - ignorance, among other factors - that women often passively accept the conditions of life that are meted out to them in the name of culture and tradition (Acsadi, and Johnson-Acsadi, 1991, p. 76).

It is due to ignorance, lack of education and the poor self-image taught to them by society, that they bear children in dark, filthy places, suffer pelvic inflammatory diseases (without questioning their source or cause), and die prematurely from the natural act of childbearing (Royston and Armstrong, 1989; United Nations, 1986). Along with the older women, who are the keepers of the culture in societies, widespread illiteracy among older men also contributes to the slow pace of change in attitudes towards women's education and self-determination.

Family Planning and Women's Health

Uncontrolled fertility aggravates many health problems for women. Too many or too closely spaced pregnancies give rise to health risks both for the mother and the infant and higher maternal and infant deaths. The health of other children in the family might also be affected, especially of the very young children who may still be dependent on maternal feeding and care (WHO, 1985).

> It is widely believed that family planning has important benefits for both maternal and child health. Although family planning can not by itself cause a substantial reduction in risk of pregnancy, the combined strategies of general fertility

reduction, abortion services, and family planning for high-risk groups might effectively address about half of all maternal mortality in the developing world. Pregnancy and delivery care have the potential for saving large numbers of lives with appropriate interventions (Winikoff and Sullivan, 1987, p. 128).

Winikoff and Sullivan are of the view that family planning can have an important impact on maternal mortality, but, by itself is not an effective approach to the problem. They suggest provision of health care as an effective means of maternal mortality prevention, along with family planning. According to them, the maximum mortality prevention might occur with a programme emphasising both family planning and health care to pregnant women. Trussell and Pebley (1984), advocate that increased use of contraception lowers the risk of maternal mortality ratio by reducing the proportion of births occurring to youngest and oldest women; by reducing the proportion of births at high parity; and by lengthening birth intervals. Because of these maternal mortality rate would further reduce as child-bearing would become less frequent. Another effect of increased contraceptive use on maternal mortality would be a reduction in the overall levels of fertility.

Trussell and Pebley further add that if women's childbearing was confined to the "prime" reproductive ages of 20-39, the maternal mortality ratio would drop by 11 per cent and the elimination of fifth and higher order births would reduce the maternal mortality ratio by about four per cent. Thus, there is distinct possibility for reducing maternal mortality through increased use of contraception. Likewise, Fortney (1987) concludes that family planning operates through three mechanisms on the level of maternal mortality; by reducing the proportion of births that are high risk; by reducing the number of unwanted pregnancies; and by reducing the total number of births.

In many countries, it would be culturally unacceptable to try and avoid or postpone the first birth after marriage, and in such societies it might be more difficult to persuade very young women to practice contraception, whereas, termination of fertility might be quite acceptable for a 35 year old woman with seven children. This is pointed out by Trussell and Pebley (1984), who advise that family planning programmes will be unlikely to reduce births to women under age 20 unless the societies in which such births are common increase the average age of marriage. In many cases, the problem is lack of access to family planning services in the developing world, especially in the rural areas and urban slums. However, the significance of the contradiction between women's stated desire to practice family planning and their reluctance to do so is enormous, and goes beyond the question of availability of services.

The ability to regulate fertility safely and effectively contributes significantly not only to the physical health of women, but also to their chance of carrying out a productive role in society (Cochrane, 1979).

For a family planning strategy to succeed, women must not only accept contraceptives, but continue to use them effectively over a prolonged period of time. However, evidence from developing countries show that both continuation rates and effectiveness of contraceptives are extremely low in many circumstances.

Factors Affecting Children's Health

Child Survival

There is widespread knowledge and awareness that mother's abilities and health are important for the child's health, as documented and evidenced in the discussion of the role of mother's education on child survival (Caldwell, 1979; Ware, 1984). Parental education is the most important influence on child survival, with mother's schooling usually having the greater impact. Child mortality declines with every additional year of a mother's education, so that even one or two years of schooling in a rural school has some impact (Caldwell and McDonald, 1981; Hobcraft, McDonald, and Rutstein, 1984). Amongst other things, a mother's education raises her skills and self-confidence; increases her exposure to information; and alters the way in which others respond to her. It also works through increasing women's autonomy (Caldwell, Reddy and Caldwell, 1983; Mosley, 1985).

When women have greater decision-making power in the household, their children's health is better cared for. Mothers' education improves child care practices and helps reduce child mortality and increases child survival. Education improves a mother's basic child-care skills, her domestic management of ill-health, efforts at preventive care and use of modern medical services The quality of care a child receives clearly affects its survival chances, which includes the kind of home-based preventive and curative care given to children and the mother's level of care in ensuring good hygiene and sanitation (Das Gupta, 1990).

Flegg (1982) showed that the level of literacy was the best indicator of low infant mortality, although the degree of equality in income and the level of medical care also played important roles. Caldwell (1986) demonstrated that low mortality was most highly correlated with the proportion of females in school a generation earlier, and that the levels of family planning practice and school attendance were also important indicators of low mortality. The association between mother's education and child mortality is slightly greater than for father's education and mortality (Clealand, 1990). Caldwell (1990) found that in Latin America, the death rate among the children of uneducated Peruvian women was almost seven times greater than among Venezuelan women with seven years of education. In Asia, the mortality among children of uneducated Nepalese women was almost 15 times greater than those of Malaysian women with seven or more years of schooling.

Maternal education is likely to produce much greater differentials in child mortality in the developing countries than in the West. In South Asia, nuclear-family residence in contrast to extended-family residence is likely to give the young mother greater control over her children's health treatment. In South India, education can produce a degree of emotional nucleation even within the extended family and can give a mother greater control over health decisions affecting her children. The improved relative survival chance of girls after five years of age in South Asia shows that increasingly children play a role in their own survival (Caldwell and Caldwell, 1987).

The World Fertility Survey showed that in the sensitive age range of 1-4 years there is excess female over male mortality throughout nearly all of North Africa, the Middle East, South Asia, and East Asia, with greater diversity in Southeast Asia and Latin America, and little or no additional danger for females only in sub-Saharan Africa (Shea 1984; Caldwell and Caldwell, 1987). Child survival depends on adequate intake of nutrients and the ability of a child to resist and recover from infections. Breast feeding contributes towards child survival by extending the period of post-partum anovulation and through post-partum abstinence and also by lengthening intervals between births.

Infant and Child Health

Infant and child mortality are important indicators of the health status of a country. Causes of infant mortality are related to immunity, health and nutritional status of pregnant mothers, the process of child birth and the care that the new born infant receives immediately after birth. A high infant mortality rate adversely affects the health of women as they are required to continue childbearing at too frequent intervals to ensure survival of the infants. In many developing countries at least half the deaths of children aged under one year occur during the first month of life and these are primarily caused by mother's poor health before and during pregnancy, and unsafe childbirth practices

(UNICEF, 1986).

In India, children below the age of five, specially in rural areas, are the worst sufferers. The death rate in the age-group 0-4 for the country as a whole is higher than that among the old people aged 50 and above (Sinha, 1990). One in ten babies born in India do not survive to celebrate their first birthday and one in three are of low birth-weight. Of the children under five years dying each year about 1.5 million die of diarrhoea, approximately 200,000 die following complications of measles, while 230,000 to 250,000 infants die within the first month of life of neonatal tetanus (UNICEF, 1984).

Infant mortality is high during the first week and 28 days after delivery. Infant deaths occurring within the first seven days of births are described as perinatal and neonatal mortality, while infant deaths beyond 28 days are called post-neonatal mortality. Neonatal mortality is attributed to prematurity, low birth weight, birth injuries, asphyxia, and congenital malformation (endogenous factors). Whereas infant deaths beyond 28 days largely arise from exogenous factors such as infections, convulsions, gastrointestinal and respiratory diseases, meningitis, infantile cirrhosis, digestive disorders, malnutrition and fevers (Mahajan, 1972; Mahadevan et al., 1986)

Mortality disparities among regions are very large during the first year of life, a vulnerable period during which unsanitary conditions and poor nutritional status are reflected in very high infant death rates in large parts of the less developed world (Pebley, 1984). There are major ethnic and cultural differentials in mortality, especially child mortality, even in the same country and with the same access to health services. It has been observed that in parts of Bihar, Madhya Pradesh, Rajasthan and Uttar Pradesh, a substantial portion of infant deaths are due to neonatal tetanus (See tables in Chapter 3). Maternal malnutrition, too, continues to be a major underlying cause of infant deaths (Sinha, 1990).

Nutritional Deficiency and Low Birth Weight

The growth and development of the foetus depend on the nutritional status of the mother. Nutritional deficiency in the mother increases her own risk and also that of the foetus. Babies born to such mothers are generally of low birth-weight and are at a higher risk of mortality than satisfactory birth weight babies (Puffer and Serrano, 1973).

In India, over 30 per cent of the new-born are of low birth-weight. Incidence of low birth-weight is high among mothers of low nutritional status (Government of India, 1984). The birth weight of a new born baby is closely linked to its chances of survival and subsequent growth and development. Low birth weight and prematurity are associated with mother's height and weight gain during pregnancy and is mainly due to insufficient food intake during pregnancy and infections such as malaria. Education of the mother has a definite positive effect on infant mortality and in every economic setting, the children of literate women have a better chance of survival than those of illiterate women (WHO, 1985b; Caldwell, 1979; Caldwell and McDonald, 1982).

In a study of three different cultural groups in India, Mahadevan et al., (1986) found that infant and childhood mortality was related to the height/ weight of the mothers. They observed that a greater number of deaths occurred at the lower levels of both height and weight distribution of the mothers, and infant and childhood mortality was also related to the nutritional status of the mother. Nutritional deficiency as a cause of the deaths of infants and children is a direct or underlying cause as well as an indirect or associated cause. Mortality risk during infancy among low birth-weight babies is nearly three times higher than that among babies of normal weight at birth (UNICEF, 1984). Maternal nutritional depletion is a serious problem for Indian women. Consequently the rate of anaemia among rural and poor urban women is very high, thus contributing towards a high infant mortality.

Causes of Death

As seen earlier, the major factors influencing infant mortality are largely related to maternal factors such as prematurity, malnutrition, asphyxia neo-natorum, delivery problems, and so on. However, water borne diseases (diarrhoea, dysentery, cholera, etc.) and air-borne diseases are also major causes of infant mortality in the developing countries of the third world.

Tetanus

Tetanus is a major killer of infants, specially of the neonates. Tetanus as a cause of neonatal death was estimated to be 39.2 per cent in rural areas and 25.3 per cent in urban areas (UNICEF, 1984). Tetanus is caused by infection of a wound. The commonest in the first month of life is due to umbilical infection. According to a survey of causes of deaths in rural areas, about 5.8 per cent of all infant deaths in 1984 were due to cord infection (Government of India, 1987). This is because of deliveries conducted by untrained birth attendants or family members, and in cases where the mothers were not immunized. In most of the home deliveries conducted by village *dais*, untrained professionals and relatives, umbilical infection is common and is caused by the use of infected instruments to cut the cord and also by fecal contaminated dressing.

The magnitude of the risk is evident from the fact that, in 1986, about 68 per cent of the deliveries in rural areas and 27 per cent in urban centres were conducted by untrained professionals and relatives (Registrar-General, 1988).

Diarrhoea

Diarrhoea is a major cause of morbidity and mortality in young children. It has been estimated that about 10 per cent of the deaths in the first year of life and about 14 per cent in ages (1-4) are due to gastroenteritis. About 50 per cent of infants and 20 per cent of pre-school children suffer from acute diarrhoeal problems. Every year, about 1.5 million children under five die because of diarrhoea, of whom 60 per cent die of dehydration (Government of India, 1988). Diarrhoea is caused by the intake of contaminated food and also because of poor personal hygiene of the mother, poor home environment and lack of a hygienic method of feeding the infant. The maximum incidence of the disease is observed during the weaning period.

Air-borne diseases

The major causes of child death in the developing countries are water-borne and air-borne diseases and fever. In addition, diseases like pneumonia and of the respiratory system, typhoid, malaria, etc., also cause infant and childhood deaths, which are preventable. Environment takes the lives of many children as they learn to move around and play around ponds and ditches, and eat and drink whatever comes their way. While maternal causes and water-borne diseases together constitute the chief causes of infant deaths, environmental factors too play a major role in affecting childhood mortality (Mahadevan et al., 1986).

Breast Feeding and Weaning

In India, several cultural practices are associated with the feeding of infants in many parts of the country. A large proportion of the population do not initiate breast feeding for one to three days. During this time period the newborn are normally given some pre-lacteal feeds to cleanse their stomach (there is a belief that the child swallows all the waste and impurities when in mothers womb). This pre-lacteal feed is believed to cleanse the infant's system. Plain water with honey, sugar or jaggery (molasses), or castor oil in some areas of Maharashtra and South India and sometimes mustard oil mixed with honey in Bangladesh and West Bengal are given to the infant as a pre-lacteal feed. The problem however, arises with the manner in which these feeds are given. Often a piece of cotton or rag is dipped in the feed and drops are squeezed into the baby's mouth. The standard of cleanliness is minimal most of the time, and it is a wonder that the infant mortality rates are not higher than reported (Visaria, 1988).

Breast feeding is universal and is normally initiated at least 24 hours after birth and more often after 48 or 72 hours. Valuable colostrum is discarded before putting infant to breast. The practice of withholding breast feeding for the first three to five days after birth deprives the child of both nourishment and the vital substances present in the colostrum that facilitate development of the child's immune response system (Visaria, 1988).

Colostrum is a yellowish colour liquid which contains immunoglobulins, lactoferrin and lysozymes which are rich in proteins, vitamins and contain antibodies and antibacterial substances which makes the infant immune to most of the diseases faced during infancy. The belief is that this yellowish colour fluid is harmful for the child's health and hence the child is seldom put to breast during the first 24 to 72 hours in most parts of rural India. Moreover, delay in initiating breast feeding may also affect the quantity of breast milk secreted because of the delay in stimulation normally provided by suckling (Wary, 1978).

Breast feeding in India is universal, prolonged and intensive without adequate nutritional support which leads to severe malnutrition of the mother. Due to repeated pregnancies and prolonged breast feeding, a majority of women suffer from anaemia, coupled with lack of sufficient nutrition (Khan et al., 1986). The practice of prolonged lactation is excellent, but is often associated with delayed introduction of supplementary food. Food supplementation usually starts after the child is 10-12 months old in most of the rural areas. Breast feeding, although beneficial in the early months, is an insufficient source of nutrients beyond the sixth month of life for the infant (Wray, 1978). Prolonged breast feeding is common in India. The duration of breast-feeding bears a relationship to the nutritional status of the child and even with the incidence of infant and child mortality. The mortality is higher for infants and children during the period when supplementary weaning foods are started.

Infant deaths during the fourth to twelfth months are mostly attributed to infant weaning practices and introduction of weaning foods or due to wrong child care practices including lack of immunisation. The mothers in the rural areas of the country tend to terminate breast-feeding mostly due to lack of milk secretion, conception and refusal of the child to be fed. These practices reveal the need for educating mothers to encourage introduction of supplementary food earlier for their infants.

In India, supplementary food is generally given after cooking. Most of the times there is no regular and fixed time for feeding the infants, it often coincides with the food timings of the adults or when the baby cries. Intermittent feeds consist of biscuits, fruits, sweets, etc. The supplementary foods given during early childhood consist mostly of cereals and pulses (Mahadevan et al, 1986).

Breast feeding provides the best nutrition for the newborn babies and protects both the nursing infant and the mother by suppressing ovulation and extending the duration of post-partum amenorrhea to a certain degree. In a non-contraceptive society child spacing is governed mainly by customs related to breast feeding and post-partum abstinence. The custom of post-partum abstinence is practiced in a traditional society because of the belief that harmful effects would be passed on to the babies through the breast milk. Breast feeding can therefore affect child survival by its role in nutrient intake, in spacing of births, and through its anti-infective properties. However, the duration of breast feeding in most countries is the longest among uneducated women who breast feed according to age-old traditions, for about one and a half years to two years. Educated mothers, even if they attend school only for some years and did not even complete primary education, wean their child earlier (Acsadi and Johnson-Acsadi, 1991; Pebley 1984).

Framework for Analysing Maternal Health

To better understand the complexities and barriers which hinder rural women's health a comprehensive framework for analysing the health status in India has been developed. The framework encompasses the socio-economic, cultural and behavioural factors that affect health and also the utilisation of services that influence health and health care behaviour. The framework was constructed by reviewing the existing framework developed by McCarthy and Maine (1992) for analysing maternal mortality, and also by reviewing the existing literature on maternal mortality, child survival, socio-economic and cultural aspects of health for women in the developing world and is also based on the data collected from the field.

One of the conclusions of the framework is that a woman's health is affected by her status in the family, housing condition, exposure to the mass-media and the village infrastructure. These are intrinsically linked with the woman's health and nutritional status, her workload, her reproductive status, awareness of and her willingness to utilise the available health services, attitude towards modern health services, health care behaviour and most significantly the cultural practices and taboos associated with pregnancy, childbirth and lactation, which frequently militate against the use of available modern health services. These immediate factors affect the outcome of pregnancy and childbirth which lead to health problems encountered either during pregnancy or after delivery and during lactation which often lead to either morbidity and mortality of the newborn and of the mother.

Most research and studies have mainly concentrated on the causes and risks of maternal mortality and its determinants like the socio-economic factors, access to health services, transportation factor, obstetric, reproductive, behavioural, demographic and biological factors, child survival and so on (Acsadi, and Johnson-Acsadi, 1991, 1986; Ojanuga, and Gilbert, 1992; Maine et al., 1987; Royston and Armstrong, 1989; Shariff, 1987; Mosley and Chen, 1984). Relatively few reports and studies however, have explicitly considered the pathways through which these diverse factors influence maternal health and morbidity. Few authors have addressed the entire process or pathways through which a host of diverse factors affect maternal health and which ultimately culminate in maternal morbidity or death. Fathalla (1987), described the "road to death" women follow, a road that starts with underlying socio-economic conditions of life and includes demographic and health service factors that lead to death. Other authors have mainly focused on the events of a pregnancy complication and factors that influence delays in seeking medical care (Thaddeus and Maine, 1990).

Although these studies and research have taken an approach to understanding the determinants of maternal mortality and morbidity, they have not presented any comprehensive models for determinants of maternal mortality or morbidity. McCarthy and Maine used these same approaches to present a comprehensive framework for analysing maternal mortality, and this framework can also be applied to study chronic maternal morbidity which results from pregnancy or childbirth. McCarthy and Maine's framework is not designed to capture the determinants of relatively minor and short duration morbidity but of the severe, long-standing serious maternal morbidity only.

They use the term "disability" in the framework to refer to chronic and severe morbidity that results from either pregnancy or childbirth; and the ultimate outcome of their framework is maternal death or disability.

Using these same approaches, an attempt has been made to present a framework for analysing the health of rural women in India. Though the framework presented is based on the McCarthy and Maine model, the model varies significantly as it deals with the health of rural women in India and focuses on the utilisation of available health care services and awareness about the available health care services, and the underlying socio-economic and cultural practices and taboos impeding use of the available services. Besides, the framework explores in-depth and in detail the cultural taboos and practices related to pregnancy, childbirth and lactation which negatively affects a woman's health. Moreover, the suggested model deals with the totality of a woman's health.

Figure 1 presents a framework for analysing the determinants of maternal mortality developed by McCarthy and Maine and includes the basic stages in the process that culminate in maternal disability or death. The framework is organised around three stages. In the event of maternal disability a sequence of outcomes follows; these outcomes are pregnancy and pregnancy-related complications. This sequence of outcomes are most directly influenced by five sets of intermediate determinants; the health status of the woman, her reproductive status; her access to health services; her health care behaviour (including her use of health services); and a set of unknown factors. Finally, a set of socio-economic and cultural background is included which is distant from a maternal death, according to McCarthy and Maine. Refer to Figure 1.

Figure 1   A framework for analysing the determinants of maternal mortality and morbidity

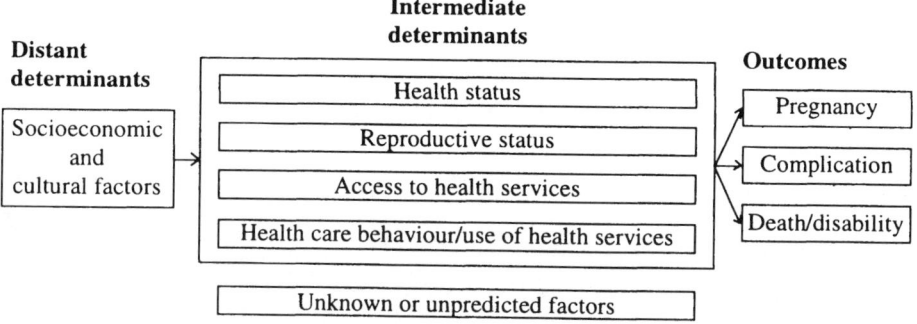

Source: (McCarthy and Maine, 1992)

McCarthy and Maine state that the socio-economic and cultural background factors are at the greatest distance from a maternal death, which is debatable. In a developing country like India, and particularly in the rural areas, the socio-economic and cultural factors play an important role in determining the well-being and health of a woman. The socio-economic and cultural factors often affect a woman's health either indirectly or directly and also influence her use of health services, her health care behaviour and attitude towards modern health care services. The non-use of the health services affects her reproductive and health status, and socio-cultural practices affect her nutritional status. Hence there is a greater need for close examination and identification of variables associated with socio-economic and cultural factors contributing towards maternal health and morbidity in India.

The cultural factors greatly influence the outcome of a mother's health status in rural India. One of the limitations of the McCarthy and Maine model is that they have placed together the socio-economic and cultural factors, and have given less importance to the cultural factors contributing towards maternal health and morbidity. However, the cultural factors associated with pregnancy, labour and delivery, and lactation play a major role and are an immediate determinant affecting maternal health in rural India. In a developing country, the socio-economic, socio-cultural and general health factors affecting maternal morbidity and mortality are much more important than the directly responsible obstetric or medical causes (Sundari, 1992).

A Framework for Analysing Maternal Health in Rural India

Figure 2 presents a detailed framework for understanding and analysing the determinants of maternal morbidity and health in rural India. The framework includes the basic and primary stages through which the outcomes are affected and a brief description of each of those stages. The framework revolves around three basic components which affect maternal health either directly or indirectly, and invariably lead to maternal morbidity which normally arises due to pregnancy, pregnancy-related complications and health problems encountered after childbirth, which contribute either towards maternal and/or infant morbidity and/or mortality.

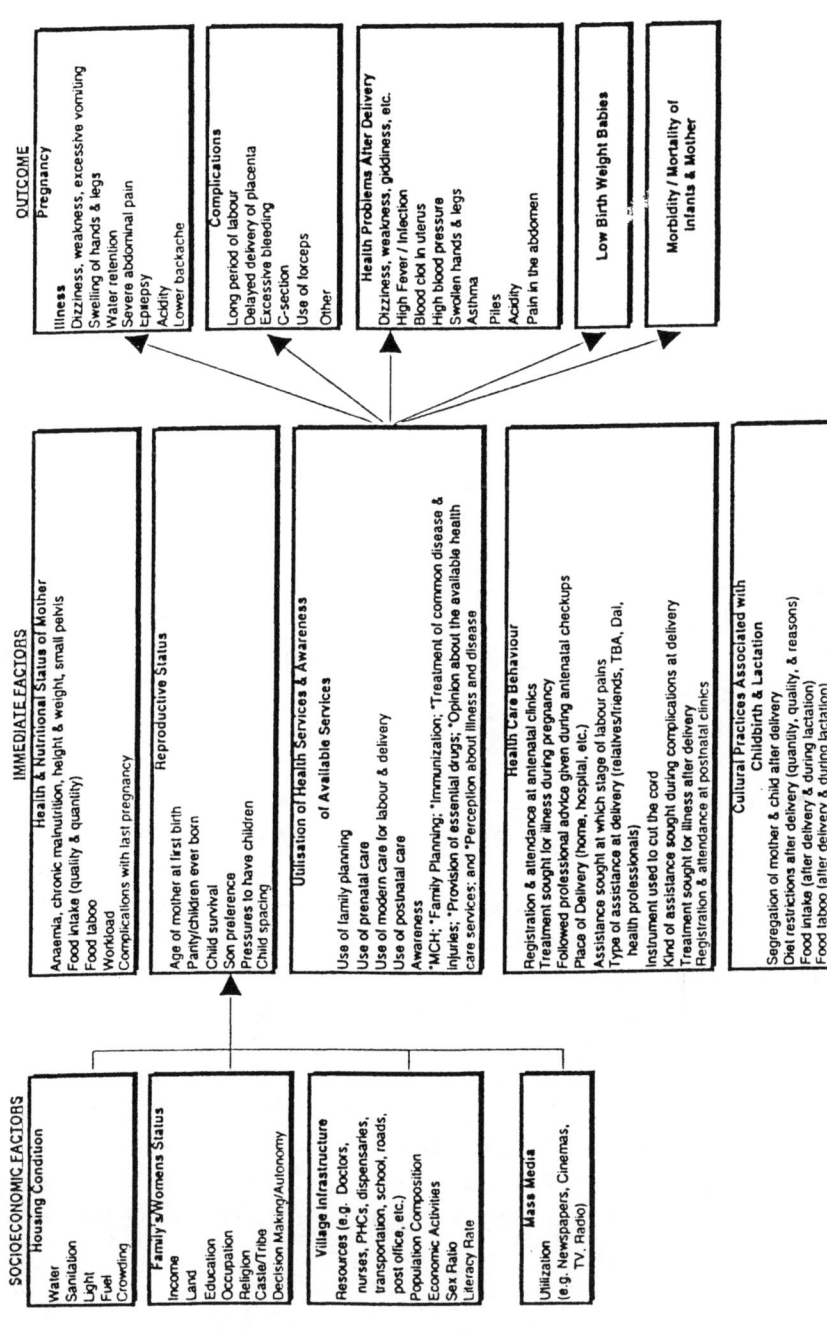

Figure 2 Framework for analysing maternal health in rural India

Socio-economic Factors Affecting Health of the Mother

Socio-economic factors play a major role in determining health status of women in India, particularly in the rural areas of the country. Differentials in maternal health status and morbidity by socio-economic status exist within countries and between urban and rural geographical locations. Socio-economic status operates at the individual, family and community level.

Figure 2 represents the indicators of socio-economic status. For women in rural India, status in the family and in the community/village is often related to their level of education, their occupation, their income or wealth, decision-making power or autonomy such as their ability to travel on their own or to make independent decisions to use health services either for themselves or their children, spending money on food and so on. Status of women is also related and linked with the caste and religious beliefs of a family. Moreover, the collective resources and wealth of the village or community they live in are also an important dimension of socio-economic status that are likely to have an influence on the health of the community or village people. The housing condition, source of water (drinking, washing, cleaning) sanitation and plumbing, source of light, fuel used for cooking and space available in the house or crowded conditions also affect maternal health adversely and these factors too operate thorough the immediate factors to influence maternal health.

Socio-economic status does not necessarily affect a woman's health directly but operates through a set of immediate determinants that affects the outcomes in the framework such as pregnancy and illness during pregnancy; complications during labour and delivery; illness after childbirth; low birth weight babies; morbidity and or mortality of the infant and of the mother. Most of the variables in the socio-economic status affect the health of women either directly or indirectly. A woman's educational attainment influences her attitude and use of modern health care, and education also makes her more assertive in using health care and changing her health care behaviour. Economic independence and education give her more autonomy in access, mobility and more power in the decision-making processes within the household with regards to her children's health and her own health. Religion too plays an important role for women in utilisation of health care and health care behaviour.

Immediate Factors Affecting Maternal Health

Health and Nutritional Status of Mother

A woman's personal health status prior to and during a pregnancy can have an important influence on her chances of developing any health problems or illness during pregnancy or having pregnancy-related complications like excessive bleeding or a long period of obstructed labour. Pre-existing health conditions that are aggravated by pregnancy and delivery are anaemia and chronic malnutrition, which often lead to haemorrhage during childbirth.

Other problems associated with pregnancy and childbirth are anaemic condition of the mother during pregnancy, a small pelvis which obstructs easy birth, heavy workload of the mother without adequate nutrition leading to premature and small, low birth weight babies. Moreover, malaria during pregnancy leads to anaemia which in turn can affect women by excessive bleeding during delivery which could lead to death of the mother (WHO, 1985b; Maine et al., 1987; Royston and Armstrong, 1987). The presence of some of these conditions may put women at a higher risk of either dying from one of the direct complications of pregnancy or they can encounter severe health problems after delivery.

Reproductive Status

The relationship between maternal age, parity, number of children ever born, close-spaced pregnancies, preference for sons, put women in a vulnerable position. The risks that a woman might become severely ill or die are often very high for very young and older women, women with no children and women with many children. Age, especially, very young age is also associated with morbidity and mortality that results from childbirth and pregnancy. Birth spacing and child survival also affect maternal health.

Utilisation of Health Services and Awareness of Available Health Services

Since the study was conducted in villages where health services were available, access to the health care centres for the study population was not a problem. But mere provision of health services does not lead to their better utilisation. 'For services to be effective women have to use them. The use of prenatal care (to diagnose either pre-existing health problems or to detect certain complications) and the use of care during and after labour and delivery (to treat complications that may arise then) are particularly important in the case of maternal mortality and morbidity. Other health care behaviours are also likely to have important influences on the outcome of pregnancy for women' (McCarthy and Maine, 1992, pp. 27). The mere existence of health services does not necessarily increase the awareness of their availability and utilisation depends upon women's perception of illness and disease and to a certain extent on the opinion of the villagers regarding the available health services.

Health Care Behaviour

Health care behaviour and attitude towards available health services are important in determining the use of the same. For services to be effective women have to register and attend the clinics (antenatal and postnatal) during pregnancy and after delivery and also use the services for labour and delivery. They should also follow the professional advice given during these clinic visits and checkups and they should be made aware so as to not ignore their well-being and put the husbands' or childs' welfare before their own. Even though a large number of women in the developing countries (especially in rural West Bengal) attend an antenatal clinic, they are shy of using the available health services for labour and delivery purposes.

Though many women face health problems after delivery, almost none of the women go for a postnatal checkup or attend a postnatal clinic. Postnatal attendance is to detect infections related to complications of delivery for both the mother and the child. It seems the concept of postnatal care has not evolved in the rural areas of India. Women tend to associate any health problems after delivery as a natural occurrence and refuse to use any health care for the same.

Cultural Practices Associated with Pregnancy, Childbirth and Lactation

Some of the cultural practices are advantageous and good for the health of the mother and the child, like breast feeding, the practice of sexual abstinence after childbirth to help space pregnancies, and so on. But there are some cultural and traditional practices that are associated with pregnancy, childbirth and lactation which are harmful to a mother's as well as the infant's health. These practices are related to nutrition and food intake in terms of quality and quantity. Both during pregnancy and after delivery and sometimes even during lactation, food taboos are observed. In some societies women are restricted to eat two meals a day and all the animal protein is cut from their diet in the event of a delivery in the best interest of the mother's and the child's health. The quality and quantity of food intake deteriorates even more so after delivery and during pregnancy too. This makes a woman more weak, anaemic and she suffers from chronic malnutrition both during pregnancy and after childbirth owing to rigid cultural practices with regards food. Therefore the newborn too suffers as a consequence of mother's deteriorating health status.

Concept of Pollution

Concepts of purity, pollution, defilement are a reflection of cultural attitudes to the body and the organisation of these attitudes into a status hierarchy (Bauer, and Karp, 1978). The cultural norms of behaviour generally presents rules concerning taboo, purity and pollution. The concept of food and hygiene can also be used as an instrument of power strategy and social stratification to emphasise the dichotomy between purity and pollution (Kramer, 1987; Woortmann, 1986). Further, Woortmann argues that the classification of food is essentially a classification of social beings in a social hierarchy.

The concept of pollution is a powerful and enduring force in Indian society and because of this the newborn and the mother are often kept separate after childbirth to keep away pollution from the other members of the family. Pollution in Indian society can be either temporary or permanent. Temporary pollution exist surrounding menstruation, contact with lower castes, births and deaths, while permanent pollution is intrinsic to the caste system and to the division of labour and is not affected by purificatory measures. For example, the washerman who washes soiled linen or the leather worker who removes and skins cattle carcasses, live in a state of permanent impurity. However, permanent pollution like temporary pollution, is a matter of degree. The Brahmin is purest among the living, but is also vulnerable to pollution by any inferior. In caste system pollution is not primarily a matter of danger to the person but has wider social implications for individuals and groups (Seymour-Smith, 1986).

Caste in India has traditionally governed not only the social, economic, and ritual lives of rural communities, but also residential patterns and other spatial relationships. Generally location and layout of village houses are determined according to their status in the local caste hierarchy. But the crucial element is segregation based on ritual purity and pollution. Ritually unclean or untouchable castes are located on the periphery of the village and only castes at similar purity levels can co-reside. Muslims are also segregated

(Mudiraj, 1973).

Douglas (1966), analyses the ritualistic props of social reality relative to pollution, cleanliness, hygiene, and the idea of dirt. Pollution powers are inherent in the structure of ideas and is a type of danger which is likely to occur except where the lines of structure are clearly defined. The notion of dirt or pollution implies a system of ordered relations, that is, the concept of pollution arises from the desire for order, and in this order, a polluting person is always in the wrong. The polluting person either develops some bad condition or simply crosses some line which should not have been crossed and this displacement releases danger for others. Pollution can be committed intentionally, but is more likely to happen unintentionally.

The sociological origin of dirt is similar to that of Durkheim's origin of deviance according to Bergesen (1978). The biological body is commonly seen as a symbol for the social body and bodily control symbolises social control. In general, homogeneity contributes to the cohesiveness of a social structure, and a polluted person is seen to be in variance to that organisation and is considered marginal, because social relations contribute to personal identity and this can be greatly threatened if those relations cease. Normally, unclear, marginal, and equivocal social situations produce ideas of power, potency, and danger. A polluted person is not necessarily guilty of social transgression, but is often condemned because of marginality. Pollution is usually activated in situations of undue proximity or excessive distancing (Douglas, 1966; Bergesen, 1978; Gomes da-Silva, and Douglas, 1984; Kramer, 1987).

Thompson (1985), argues that 'the nexus of beliefs connected with women's pollution and other mystical powers encourages women to subordinate their interests to men's'. In traditional Hindu village society, women are seen as having the power to pollute men. Female sexuality is associated with pollution because of their biology and other circumstances. When associated with pollution, women are perceived as being in danger as well as endangering others.

In a study in southern India, Deliege (1992), found that the villagers perceived demonic possession as a punishment for ritual pollution, that is, negligence of ritual purity rules. Moreover, the main victims of demonic possessions are usually women, and they are possessed due to pollution related to sexuality and reproduction. In certain societies specific persons become temporarily impure due to menstruation or a birth and death in the family and are thus unable to perform certain duties. The length of incapacitation varies according to the person's occupational class, place of residence and socio-economic status in the community (Mines, 1989).

The Beta Israel (Falashas), a Jewish group from Ethiopia, view menstruation, circumcision, excision and infibulation of newborn girls, deaths, and contact with outsiders, as sources of pollution (Semi, 1985). Likewise, the Huli people of Papua New Guinea, believe that women who have just given birth or who are also experiencing menopause can have destructive influence upon men (Frankel, 1980). The notions of ritual purity and pollution are normally limited to physical objects, including space (Madan, 1985).

Paige and Paige (1981), argues that rituals are instituted by males to gain political and economic control of society through control of women's reproductive power. While Balzer (1981), is of the view that conflicting norms of male dominance and female independence can encourage pollution beliefs. Further, Lawerence (1982), argues that women's behaviour can be explained not by reference to assumptions of male dominance over women, but to women's conscious choice of modes of behaviour reflecting strategic goals important to their own perceived self-interest. The author stresses that women are the principal actors in maintaining the menstrual taboo because it allows them to control certain social interactions outside the household. Ultimately women's behaviour related to the menstrual taboo is viewed as embedded within the complexity of the social relations and values that surround them, rather than as a simple function of pollution concepts.

On the ritual front of purity and pollution, a double standard has emerged according to Atal (1978). The upper castes, while visiting urban centres, do not rigidly observe the rules of social and ritual distance, but back in the village, they conform to caste norms, beliefs and practice taboos relating to purity, pollution and danger.

These cultural practices put the mother in a disadvantageous position and make her vulnerable to all kinds of infections and illness which she is unable to ward off because of her weak immune system. Thus the chances are high for the mother to fall ill during pregnancy or after childbirth because of repeated insults to her health.

Outcomes

Illness

This outcome is the direct result of deteriorating maternal health and maternal morbidity due to repeated closely spaced pregnancies in the extreme age groups.

In addition, cultural and social pressures to marry early and have children immediately after marriage, and preference for sons to continue the patrilineal lineage affects women's health irreparably. Women in rural areas of India enter into marriage and embark on a reproductive career ill-prepared, without any adequate education, lack of awareness, complete ignorance in most cases, and experience a host of problems during pregnancy. 'It is important to include pregnancy as the starting point of the sequence of outcomes leading to maternal morbidity, because the risk of pregnancy varies considerably from woman to woman, and because pregnancy rates vary so greatly among different groups of women' (McCarthy and Maine, 1992).

Complications

This outcome is also the result of repeated insults to a woman's health and to her reproductive status. Because of these constant onslaughts rural women face difficulties during labour and delivery and also during the post-partum period. Many women prior to pregnancy have a pre-existing medical condition or history that is made worse by the pregnancy and delivery. The long and prolonged period of obstructed labour, excessive bleeding often leading to haemorrhage, hypertension, delayed delivery of placenta and ruptured uterus are the major causes of delivery-related complications (WHO, 1985b; Maine et al., 1987).

Postpartum Health Problems

The most common form of postpartum health problems are high fever and infection, weakness, dizziness, swollen hands and legs, blood clot in the uterus and so on, because of malnutrition and inadequate food intake, lack of prenatal care etc.

Low Birth Weight Babies

This outcome is because of maternal health and nutritional status, order of birth, parity, age of the mother, illness during pregnancy, workload and so on, as previously discussed.

Morbidity and Mortality of Infants and Mothers

The final outcome of the framework is either morbidity and/or mortality of the infant and the mother due to a host of direct and indirect factors such as the socio-economic, socio-cultural factors, the obstetric or medical factors and so on.

The framework has tried to explain the pathways through which a mother's health is affected in rural India. The health of a mother can be affected because of a host of direct and indirect factors contributing towards their already dismal health status. The framework presented here is not an exhaustive one, further research and studies could be conducted on the basis of this framework. The present framework can further be modified to study the health of women in other cultural contexts and can also be applied to study child survival and children's health and how maternal factors affect children's health. This model can be relevant and significant for further theorisation in the area of maternal and child health to validate the assumptions made in reference to the intricate relationship between cultural and traditional factors affecting maternal health. It can also be used as a methodological guideline for further studies and can also act as a guide for policy and programme development in the area of maternal health.

Perspectives on Health in India

Profiles of the four villages in which four hundred households were surveyed are presented here. This chapter introduces in considerable detail the geographical location, physical setting, demographic characteristics, socio-economic conditions, and also the health care perception, behaviour, and utilisation. In addition, general health situation of India and the state of West Bengal is also presented. Details of the mortality and fertility situation in the country and major states of India is also presented.

A Thumbnail Sketch of the Research Sites

Village Motipur (District Puruliya)

Location of the study area
The district of Puruliya lies to the west of Calcutta, and is the westernmost district of the state of West Bengal. It is about 220 kilometres from the Bay of Bengal and the Hugli estuary. The study was conducted in a village of this district called Motipur, administered by the Block headquarters of Hura police station. The village is about 34 km. from the nearest town, and is not connected by either a national/state highway or railway. The bus-stop is at Hura, which is 5 km. from the village. The road leading to the village from the bus-stop is an unsurfaced and pebbled pathway.

Puruliya is predominantly an agricultural district. According to the 1981 census, 75.19 per cent of the total workers of the district were dependent on agriculture (that is, cultivators and agricultural labourers). Rice is the main cultivated crop, followed by wheat and pulses.

Although agriculture is the chief source of livelihood the irrigation facilities in the district are far from satisfactory. The district is characterised by the presence of large waste lands and has a gently undulating topography with hillocks of hard rocks. Even though a large number of rivulets originate in the district itself, owing to the natural topography, these rivers and rivulets offer few possibilities for irrigation. Irrigation in the district is provided by tanks and '*bundhs*' (a type of water reservoir) from accumulation of runoff water. The accumulation of water in the tanks and the *bundhs* depends only on rainfall. The reservoirs mostly dry up during the summer months. Irrigation using wells covers but a portion of the total cultivable land.

According to the 1981 census only 11.44 per cent of the total cultivable land area of the district is irrigated. The sources of irrigation in Motipur are by means of wells (1.21 hectare) and tanks (40.47 hectare). About 306.75 hectares of land is unirrigated, and the area not available for cultivation is 215.71 hectares, cultivable waste (including orchards and groves) is approximately 131.52 hectares.

The staple diet in this area is rice, followed by wheat. The village does not have any electricity, but the Block headquarters has a power supply. The forest area surrounding this village is approximately 13.76 hectares. According to the 1981 census the total land area of Motipur is 709.02 hectare.

Physical setting
The bus-stop is close to the police station and the Block Primary Health Centre (BPHC) on the main road, which is also the market place of the town. Though the road is made of tar, it is full of big potholes. On both sides of the main road are concrete buildings housing government offices, schools, different shops and restaurants. To reach the village one has to depend on cycle-rickshaws or walk the distance of 5 km. The main road of the Block connects with the district town of Puruliya 34 km. away. The main road bifurcates, one leading to the district town and the other to the village proper. On the way to the village is the cinema hall. There are some huts close to the cinema hall on both sides of the pathway.

The Block Development Office (BDO) is a huge complex situated a little further on from the cinema hall. The village is some 2 km. from the BDO, with a dusty pathway leading into the village. The village is relatively quiet in the mornings except for some stray goats and children playing in the dust and soil. Everybody else is engaged in their daily chores. The village is poor (all the huts are made of mud and are thatched), the housing compounds/yards are kept very clean by constant sweeping and coating the courtyard with cow-dung and water, so that the dust cannot be carried into the house. The huts are neat and clean and tiny, but very dark and gloomy inside.

In the evenings, the village is alive with the singing and dancing of the tribal men and women. Since the village is devoid of any electricity, it is very dark and eerie during the evenings. Strangers are not at all welcome in the village and they are looked upon with suspicion. Both men and women are reluctant to talk to strangers about anything to do with their lifestyles. For every little thing they need, they have to cover the distance of 5 km. to the Block headquarters. The village seems to be very detached from the real world and also from the Block. This village is a world unto itself.

The population

The total population of the village is 1318 according to the 1981 census, out of which 406 persons are literate (31%). The village is almost entirely inhabited by tribals and scheduled castes (68%), and there are a total of 228 households in this village. The demographic features of the village population are as follows; and it has been observed that some of the villagers engage in more than one kind of economic activity in the surveyed village.

Population	Total	Male	Female
	1318	703	615
(i) General	454	250	204
(ii) Scheduled Castes	39	19	20
(iii) Scheduled Tribes	825	434	391
Economic Activities			
(i) Main Workers	375	267	108
(ii) Cultivators	226	212	14
(iii) Agricultural Labourers	103	10	93
(iv) Household Industry	04	04	...
(v) Other Workers	42	41	01
(vi) Marginal Workers	225	87	138
(vii) Non-Workers	718	349	369
Literate	406	333	73

Amenities Available	
(i) Educational	P(2) [Grades I-IV]
	H [Grades IX-X]
(ii) Medical	(- 5 km.) away
(iii) Drinking Water (potable)	W, TW (Well and Tube-well)
(iv) Post and Telegraph	(- 5 km.) away
(v) Day or Days of the Market, if any	(- 5 km.) away
(vi) Communication Hura (Bus-Stop)	(- 5 km.)
(vii) Approach to Village	KR (Kuccha Road) Pathway
(viii) Nearest Town and distance in Km.	Puruliya 34 km.

(*Source:* District Census Handbook, District Puruliya, 1981)

Facilities and amenities

Almost all the facilities and amenities are available surrounding the police station and the Block headquarters. The bus-stop is close to the market and the police station. The Block Primary Health Centre (BPHC) is next to the police station. Besides the BPHC there is an Animal Husbandry and Veterinary Hospital in the area. There are several co-operatives in this area to aid the villagers and especially the tribals and other scheduled caste population to sell their produce at a fair price at the government controlled co-operatives. The Block Development Office (BDO) and the 'Gram Panchayat Office' (elected local self government – the current political party holding office is the Communist Party of India – Marxist) is much closer to the village.

The other amenities/facilities available in this area are a post office, a revenue office, a ration shop (where essential supplies and food can be purchased at government controlled rates), a state bank (where agricultural loans and other loans can be obtained for the unemployed youth).

Most villages in this area are under the Integrated Child Development Scheme Programme (ICDS), which is run by the government for the benefit of pregnant women, infants and children under the age of five. The ICDS project has a sponsored 'Anganwadi Centre' (Day Care Centre) in the village for babies and pregnant and lactating women, where a supplementary and balanced diet is given to both expectant and lactating mothers and the children. The 'Anganwadi Centre' monitors the growth of the babies, immunises them against infectious diseases and also serves as a referral service.

An Integrated Rural Development Project (IRDP) is also run in the area by the Government of India, which basically stresses new methods of farming. Besides there is a government run farm in the area which employs some of the tribals and other people from the village. To assist in the IRDP project, an Office of the Agricultural Development Officer has been created to monitor the progress of the IRDP programme.

Block Hura also has a Forest Department, Block Land and a Land Reform Office (State government policy to redistribute land to the landless, agricultural labourers and to the economically and other backward classes). Within the 5 km. distance there are two primary schools (Grades 1-4), a high school and a college which is 3 km. away from the Block headquarters.

Households surveyed
To study the maternal and child health care practices besides the health care utilisation and perception, 100 households were chosen at random with at least one eligible woman in each household in the reproductive age between 13-49 years. All the households studied were tribals in this village.

Housing condition
The main source of drinking water for 69 per cent of the households surveyed is the public hand-pump (deep bore well). Around 68 per cent of the households use the pond or lake for bathing and washing. About 91 per cent of the households use kerosene lamps as the source of lighting. Electricity is provided only for agricultural purposes. A majority of the surveyed households (99%) use firewood for cooking, and 63 per cent use their verandah as a kitchen. Most of the surveyed houses have one (38%) to two (42%) rooms on an average. A majority of the village population and the households surveyed (98%) do not have any toilet/latrine facilities.

Land holdings and cultivation
Almost all the landless labourers and the other economically backward classes and the tribals of this area were given 0.133 acre of land per family by the Communist State government under their 'Land Reform Scheme'. This scheme was to provide an opportunity for these under-privileged people to live a life with dignity and not depend on the big land owners for jobs. But this gesture of the State government seems to be futile because nearly all the tribals and other scheduled caste people of this village do work as agricultural labourers or manual labourers to supplement their income and subsistence.

Most of the villagers own some kind of agricultural land (71%) with 93 per cent of the surveyed population being solely dependent on rain for irrigation. Of those who do own some kind of agricultural land, almost everybody (70%) grows only rice. Most of the agricultural work in the fields is done by the family members (61%), and whatever is grown is just enough for their own subsistence, they rarely have extra to sell at the co-operatives which have been especially set up for the benefit of the tribals and other tribal villages to safeguard them against middlemen.

Besides owning agricultural land, most of the villagers keep cattle and livestock to supplement their subsistence. Normally they keep cows and goats for milk, hens and ducks for eggs and meat, and bullocks for ploughing their fields. About 71 per cent of the households own some kind of livestock. They generally keep the cattle outside the house, in their household compound/yard at night and keep the hens, ducks, and goats inside the house at night.

Assets

As compared to the other study villages, the economic status of village Motipur, is quite poor. Only about 23 per cent of the household surveyed owned either a clock or a wrist-watch. Around 24 per cent owned a radio/transistor. The basic means of transportation in this area are bicycles (45%) and bullock-carts (4%), followed by public transportation which is 5 km. from the village.

Family type, composition, occupation and income

Nuclear families seem to be the norm in all the surveyed villages. In village Motipur, too, more than half the households surveyed were nuclear, and the rest were extended or joint family system The nuclear families normally consisted of three to four children. Amongst the 102 households surveyed, there were 281 males to 240 females (total population of the survey was 521), out of which 181 were literate (35%), and 176 persons (34%) had some form of schooling. Family size in the village varied from four to seven members (68%). The desired family size of this village is that of two boys and two girls, or three boys and one girl.

An overwhelming 43 per cent of the women surveyed worked outside homes as manual/agricultural labourers, in farming and cultivation and a few had some small household based industry/business of their own to run. The remaining were "housewives". Hence, almost all the women surveyed have dual roles to play, both within and outside the house. A tribal woman's normal day begins before sunrise and ends long after sunset. She does all the household chores of cooking, cleaning, washing, caring for children, sick and elderly, fetching water, firewood, feeding the family members, children and also the cattle, cleaning the cattle-shed, bearing and rearing children, working as a labourer and also working in the family's own fields during harvesting and sowing seasons, threshing and husking paddy or wheat, preparing puffed rice and rice crisps for home consumption. Whereas in comparison only 38 per cent men till their land and 41 per cent work as labourers, 11 per cent run their own small scale business and a further 10 per cent are employed in service. The men do not help in the house as these are considered to be strictly women's chores and duties.

The total monthly income of the majority of the surveyed households

(55%), was very low (Rupees 100-500). 35 per cent were in the range of Rs. 501-1000, and 8 per cent belonged in the range of Rs. 1001-2500, and a mere two per cent were in the category of Rs. 2501-10,000 (US$ 1 = 35.85 Rs.). For details please see table 4.9 in Chapter 4.

Health care utilisation and perception
Even though the Primary Health Care (PHC) Centre is located at a distance of 5 km. from the village, the villagers use it frequently (mostly a last resort). Medical pluralism exists to some extent in all the four villages surveyed, but it is more so in Motipur. The surveyed population of village Motipur have immense faith in traditional healers, quacks, black magic and witch-craft. They have *Shamans*, referred to as *Ojha*, in the local dialect of the tribals living in the village. Hence, for any kind of ailment or health related problems they consult the *Ojha* first, and wait for two-three days for results and if the problem still persists they consult the village quack and then lastly visit the PHC or the government hospital for treatment. Almost 100 per cent of the surveyed population had used the facilities of the PHC at some point of time or other for minor ailments like coughs and colds, fever, influenza, dysentery and diarrhoea.

About 52 per cent of the surveyed population complained that they had some problem in seeking treatment from the health centre. The most common complaint was that medicines were never available (40%). Only about 40 per cent of the surveyed population consulted with a trained private practitioner/ doctor for major ailments. The opinion of the villagers regarding the PHC was 'fair' (40%), and about 28 per cent of the villagers felt that it was 'bad' and 26 per cent thought that the PHC was giving a 'satisfactory' service (Refer to Table No. 5.5 in Chapter 5).

The surveyed population used the PHC to cure illness and to get relief from diseases and other ailments. Moreover, after experimenting with alternative medicines they ultimately visit the PHC for treatment and cure. Some of the heads of household complained that the health centre doctors preferred to see patients during their spare time in their private chambers. According to these villagers the treatment by the same PHC doctors was better at their private clinic than at the PHC.

In case of any illness in the family the head of the family or in the absence of the head, any elderly relative makes the decision regarding the type of treatment to be sought for adult males and females suffering from illness. In case of adult females, more often than not, traditional home remedies are administered, or depending on the type of ailment, either the services of the *Ojha* or the village quack are utilised. But 90 per cent of the surveyed females reported that they visit the PHC, as compared to 95 per cent males.

The study populations' perception regarding major and minor common illness is based on their own personal experience or on the experience of their kith and kin. Accordingly they classified tuberculosis (30%); cholera (29%); dysentery and diarrhoea (86%) and malaria (41%) as major common ailments. A majority of these people did not know anything about blood pressure, diabetes, bronchitis, infections, or pneumonia. Headaches (70%), cough and cold (70%), fever (81%) and so on were perceived as minor ailments, and they consulted with their village quacks for these ailments, and if it persisted for long they visited the PHC for cure and relief from the ailment. A majority of the women surveyed had knowledge about the services available from the PHC, like the provision of family planning services (79%), maternal and child health services (81%), immunisation against infectious diseases and injuries (66%), but about 68 per cent of the surveyed women and men did not know that the health centre also provided essential drugs.

Village Kapgari (District Medinipur)

Location of the study area
The district of Medinipur lies to the far south-west of Calcutta and is about 184 km. from the city of Calcutta. The study was conducted in a village of this district called Kapgari, which is under the sub-divisional town of Jhargram and is administered by the Block headquarters of Jamboni police station. The village is about 24 km. from the sub-divisional town, and is about 8 km. away from the nearest railway station and 2 km. off the national highway. The road leading into the village from the main road is semi- asphalt.

Physical setting
Village Kapgari is 18 km. from the sub-divisional town of Jhargram, and the road that leads into the village from the main road, which is a national and state highway, is a good 2 km. inside. The village can be reached from the highway either by bullock carts, bicycles or foot, as the bus service into the village is only four times a day. The road leading into the village is made of tar, but in some places it resembles a dusty track. On both sides of the road are the paddy fields and tall coconut and palm trees. At the entrance to the village are tall bamboo and other shrubs making a canopy overhead which screens one from the strong sun. As one approaches the village, there is a sense of peace and quiet and stillness in the air. The approach road to the village is

most of the time shaded from the strong sun by tall bamboo's and other shrubs and bushes. On the main road of the village there are tiny little shops and tea-stalls, a chemist, a cycle repair shop, and other grocery and stationery stores. In all there are about a dozen or so shops.

The schools, hostel, post office, bank, Panchayat Office (Communist Party of India - Marxist), are all located close to the main road. The college is close to the other end of the village where a stream flows and divides the paddy fields of village Kapgari and the next village. There is a mango orchard next to the college grounds and the teachers' living quarters are also in this stretch of the village. At the other end of the village is the Primary Health Care Centre (PHC), where there are no residential houses. Next to the PHC is the Krishi Vigyan Kendra (KVK) Agricultural Research Centre, and Seva Bharati (Social Welfare Office). The land here is almost barren except for the tall eucalyptus planted in front of the research centre and the welfare office and PHC by the KVK. Behind the KVK is the mango, lemon and orange orchards sponsored by the KVK's agricultural research centre. There is poultry in the compound of the KVK and a dairy.

The Youth Club is situated right in the middle of a big field close to the PHC. The ground is bordered by eucalyptus plantations. Where the PHC's boundary ends, a government dam begins and on the other side of the dam, the tribals of this area live. The road leading into the village proper is just off the main road, where the tiny shops are located. The road is dusty and sandy. There is not much going on in the village unless there are religious festivals. In general the village is very quiet.

The population
According to the 1981 census the total land area of the village is 150.02 hectare, and the total population of the village is 1368 out of which 809 persons are literate (59%), and there are a total number of 212 households in the village. There is a Primary Health Centre in the village. The demographic features of the village population are as follows; and it has been observed that some of the villagers engage in more than one kind of economic activity in the surveyed village.

Population	Total	Male	Female
	1368	792	576
(i) General	1116	650	466
(ii) Scheduled Caste	132	87	45
(iii) Scheduled Tribe	120	55	65
Economic Activities			
(i) Main Workers	342	313	29
(ii) Cultivators	156	155	01
(iii) Agricultural Labourers	79	62	17
(iv) Household Industry	07	07	...
(v) Other Workers	100	89	11
(vi) Marginal Workers	22	01	21
(vii)Non-Workers	1004	478	526
Literate	809	580	229

(*Source*: District Census Handbook, District Medinipur, 1981).

Amenities Available

(i) Educational	PM (Grades I-VIII); H(Grades IX-X)
	PUC (Grades XI-XII)
	C (College of Arts, Sc. and Com.)
(ii) Medical	HC (Health Centre)
(iii) Drinking Water (potable)	W (Well)
(iv) Post and Telegraph	P.O. (Post Office)
(v) Day or Days of the Market, if any	(5-10 km.) away
(vi) Communication	BS (Bus-Stop)
(vii) Approach to Village	PR (Pukka Road); KR (Kuccha Road)
(viii) Nearest Town and distance in Km.	Jhargram 24 km.

(*Source*: Survey data, 1993)

Facilities and amenities

The village also has various administrative and welfare institutions for the surrounding villages besides the Primary Health Care Centre and the Veterinary Aid Centre. The other amenities/facilities available in the village are a post office, a revenue office, a ration shop (where essential supplies and food can be purchased at the fixed rate set by the state government), a state owned bank (where agricultural loans and other loans for starting small businesses can be obtained).

The Integrated Child Development Scheme Program (ICDS) is run in the village by the government for the benefit of pregnant women, infants and children under the age of five. The ICDS project has sponsored two 'Anganwadi Centres' for babies and pregnant women, where a supplementary and balanced diet is given both to the expectant mothers and the children. These centres also monitor the growth of the babies, immunise them against infectious diseases and provide a referral service. The project also runs a Crèche in the village.

The village boasts a College of Arts, Science and Commerce, besides the Primary, Middle, Secondary, and a Higher Secondary school, as well as a kindergarten for children under the age of five years. There is also a youth club (Kapgari Kishore Sangha) which organises various activities but it is only for males. There is a bus-stop as children and youth from nearby villages attend schools and college in this village, as they are the only ones within 24 km.

Households surveyed
Out of the 100 households studied, 84 percent were Hindus and 16 per cent were Muslims.

Housing condition
Almost 90 per cent of the houses in this village are made of earth with thatch roof and mud walls and floors. The main source of drinking water for the majority of the village population (58% of surveyed households) is the public well. Almost 75 per cent of the households use the pond or lake for washing and bathing. About 52 per cent of the households have illegally tapped into the electric power supply meant for agricultural and irrigation purposes. The majority of households (91%) use firewood for cooking, and 67 per cent of the households use their verandah as a kitchen. The houses have generally one (36%) or two (42%) rooms. Almost 88 per cent of the population do not have any toilet/latrine facility.

Land holdings and cultivation
Most of the villagers own some kind of agricultural land (70%) but are solely dependent on rain for irrigation. Of those who do own agricultural land, about 58 per cent grow only rice and very few grow other vegetables, potatoes, mustard and wheat. Most of the agricultural work in the fields is done by family members, and whatever is grown is just enough for their subsistence. Besides owning agricultural land, most of the villagers keep some kind of cattle and livestock to supplement their subsistence farming. About 77 per cent of the population own livestock. They generally keep the cattle outside

the house in cattle-sheds at night and keep the hens, ducks, and goats inside the house at night.

Assets

The economic status of the village is quite healthy as 50 per cent of the population own either a clock or a wrist-watch and 51 per cent own a radio/ transistor, while about 6 per cent own a television set, and 19 per cent own electric fans. The main means of transportation are bicycles (74%), bullock-carts (22%), and public transport. The Social Welfare Office and the Agricultural Research Centre have their own vehicles which are used by the villagers during any sort of emergency.

Family type, composition, occupation and income

More than half of the households surveyed were nuclear, and the rest were either joint or extended families. In the nuclear families there were normally three to four children. In the population surveyed, that is, 100 households, there were 307 males to 260 females (total population of the survey was 567), out of which 323 were literate (57%), and 307 people (54%) had some form of schooling. Family size in the village varied from four to seven members (71%). The most common preferred family composition of this village is two boys and two girls or three boys and one girl.

The overwhelming majority of the women surveyed (96%) took on the dual roles of being a housewife and farming the land. They do all the household chores as well as helping out during the harvesting and sowing seasons. They also thresh paddy or wheat, and prepare puffed rice for home consumption and also for selling. In comparison only 42 per cent of the males farm their land. 27 per cent of the surveyed village males work in various government jobs within the village, 35 per cent have their own small businesses and 22 per cent are labourers. Total monthly income varied from a low of Rupees 100-500 (29%) to a high of Rupees 5500 (1%). But most of the people were within the bracket of Rupees 100-1000 (US$ 1=35.85 Rupees). See table 4.9 in Chapter 4.

Health care utilisation and perception

Since the village has a Primary Health Care Centre, the villagers are aware of its services and use it very frequently (81%) for minor ailments like headaches, coughs and colds, cuts and wounds and so on. Most of the villagers (60%) complained that they had faced some problem or the other in seeking treatment from the health centre. The most common complaint was that the medicines were never available and more often than not the doctor was missing.

A majority (74%) of the population consulted with a trained private practitioner/doctor for major ailments. The opinion of the villagers regarding the PHC was 'bad' (40%). Only 11 per cent of the population felt that it was 'satisfactory' and 31 per cent said that the PHC was 'fair'. The people still continue to use the PHC because it is easily accessible and free. But many believe that since the PHC is free, the treatment is not good enough to cure the ailments. Some villagers also feel that for any kind of ailment the PHC staff and personnel always give the same kind of medicines/medications (See Table No. 5.5 in Chapter 5).

In case of illness in the family the head of the family decides regarding the type of treatment to be sought in case of adult males and females. From the survey data it has been found that in both cases the patient is taken to the health centre (64% in case of females and 66% in case of the males). But women tried home remedies first in a few stray cases (4%), and also preferred to consult with a private doctor at home.

In the study population the perception of major and minor common illness is based on their personal experience or experience of their kith and kin. Accordingly they classified tuberculosis (53%); cholera (62%); dysentery and diarrhoea (88%) and malaria (49%) as major common illnesses. A majority of them did not know about illness such as diabetes, blood pressure, bronchitis or pneumonia and so on.

Headaches (64%), coughs and colds (83%), and fever (68%) were perceived by the majority as minor ailments which did not need any kind of treatment. They felt that these ailments normally cured themselves without any medication after a certain period of time. But surprisingly enough 61 per cent sought treatment for fever and only 41 per cent for dysentery and diarrhoea. The reason behind seeking treatment in case of fever may be the easy accessibility of the health centre and moreover, the villagers do not have to pay anything for consultation and medication at the health centre. Whereas in case of dysentery and diarrhoea they have to buy the saline from the pharmacy as invariably saline is not available at the village PHCs.

Village Santoshpur (District Murshidabad)

Location of the study area

The district of Murshidabad is a triangular tract, its apex verging on the north-western extremity of the state. The district lies to the north of Calcutta city and is 232 km. from the centre of the city. The study was conducted in a village of this district called Santoshpur, which is administered by the Block headquarters of Sagardighi police station. The village is about 16 km. from the nearest town, and is well connected with a network of national and state highways and bus services to important towns, besides a railway station. Moreover, the bullock carts play a very prominent part in the economic life of the people of the village and the district. In the rural areas this is the most economical means of transportation for carrying goods and passengers as well. The road leading into the village, which is 18 km. from the state highway, is made of tar and is surfaced.

The district is located centrally in the lower Ganges valley and is prone to sudden flash floods during the monsoons as Murshidabad is interspersed by numerous rivers. The district on the eastern side of river Bhagirathi is low lying and alluvial with a humid climate and fertile soil, whereas on the western side, the surface is high and undulating and the soil is hard clay and the climate is much drier.

Agriculture plays a major and vital role in the economy of the district. According to the 1981 census 69 per cent of the total workers of the district were engaged in agricultural pursuits. Although agriculture plays a pivotal role in the village economy, there is no available means of irrigation in the area. Unirrigated land area accounts for 74.87 hectares. The area not available for cultivation is 8.09 hectares, whereas cultivable waste (including orchards and groves) is about 10.12 hectares. According to the 1981 census the total land area of the village Santoshpur is 93.08 hectares. The staple diet of the area is rice and wheat. The village has electricity. Sericulture industry (Silk-worm breeding and the production of raw silk) is the principal agro-based rural industry of the district. Another major industry in the district is that of ivory carving, which is an important cottage industry.

Physical setting
The village of Santoshpur is about 18 km. from the main road which is also a State highway. The village can be reached through the midst of picturesque and emerald green paddy fields, coconut, palm and date trees and an abundance of ponds scattered at regular intervals. Next to the Block Primary Health Centre (BPHC) of Sagardighi is the bus-stop. From the main road of Block Sagardighi a dusty and beaten track leads into the village proper. The village is lacking any activity as it is mainly residential. All the activity and noise are concentrated on the main road that belongs to the Block Sagardighi. The main road from the bus-stop leading towards the marketplace and the railway station resembles a small satellite town full of people, mainly men, busy with their work, or gathered in small groups at tiny tea-stalls and roadside cafes discussing politics,

or the day's football match between the village high school and the neighbouring village school, or cricket!

The market area is full of hawkers, selling everything from fruits to meat. Small stationery stores, grocers, chemists, a homeopathic dispensary, allopathic clinics, cycle repair shops, snack bars, cloth merchants, a hardware store, co-operative stores and offices are all located on this main road or the square. The bank, police station, schools, post-office, are also located in this area of the main road. The main road ends abruptly at the railway station of Sagardighi, and on the other side of the railway station is another village. The Block square also has a privately owned Video Parlour, where the latest films are screened, and which displays huge posters advertising the film to be shown that week. The main road is busy from 0500 hours in the morning until 1800 hours. In almost all the villages of the State of West Bengal the day begins early and ends early.

The population

Murshidabad is a predominantly Muslim district and the surveyed population of the village Santoshpur too, is predominantly Muslim (79%). Of the remaining 21 per cent of the surveyed population, 2 per cent are Scheduled Tribes, and 12 per cent belong to Scheduled Castes. The remaining seven per cent are mainly Hindu Kayasthas.

Population	Total	Male	Female
	876	430	446
(i) General	837	414	423
(ii) Scheduled Castes	29	11	18
(iii) Scheduled Tribes	10	05	05
Economic Activities			
(i) Main Workers	258	254	04
(ii) Cultivators	110	110	...
(iii) Agricultural Labourers	135	131	04
(iv) Household Industry	...	...	...
(v) Other Workers	13	13	...
(vi) Marginal Workers	...	...	...
(vii) Non-Workers	618	176	442
Literate	88	73	15
Amenities Available			
(i) Educational	P, M (grades 1-8)		
(ii) Medical	BPHC		
(iii) Drinking Water (Potable)	W, TW (Well and Tube-well)		
(iv) Post and Telegraph	PO (Post Office)		
(v) Day or Days of the Market, if any	(- 2 km. away)		
(vi) Communication	BS (Bus-Stop) and Rly.Stn.		
(vii) Approach to Village	PR (Pukka Road); R(Kuccha Road)		
(viii) Nearest Town and distance in km.	Raghunathganj 16 km. & Bahrampur 32 km.		

(*Source*: District Census Handbook, District Murshidabad, 1981).

The total population of the village is 876 out of which 88 persons are literate (10%), according to the 1981 census. The village is almost entirely inhabited by Muslims, and there are a total of 152 households in this village. The Primary Health Centre is located at the Sagardighi Block which is very close to the village. The demographic features of the village population are as follows; and it has been observed that some of the villagers engage in more than one kind of economic activity in the surveyed village.

Facilities and amenities
Village Santoshpur is located right next to the Block headquarters of Sagardighi and has quite a few administrative and welfare institutions. The Primary Health Centre (PHC), which is also referred to as the Block Primary Health Centre (BPHC) is a relatively new complex built two years ago as the old PHC did not have any bed facilities, whereas the new complex has a bed capacity of 30. The Block also has a Veterinary Hospital.

The other amenities and facilities which are available in the village and the Block are a post and telegraph office, a revenue office, a ration shop (for essential food stuffs and other basic necessities at government controlled prices), and a Co-operative Control Shop, a state bank (which provides loans for agricultural purposes, animal husbandry and other small-scale businesses).

The village and the Block are situated in such a way that a majority of the bus routes pass through this village connecting it with the major towns and cities of the district. The Block also has a railway station which connects to the main town of Bahrampur in the district and also to the neighbouring districts. The Block and the village also has a Primary School (grades 1-4), Middle School (grades 5-8), Secondary School (grades 9-10) and a Higher Secondary School (grades 11-12), but for the tertiary level education the villagers have to either attend the colleges at Raghunathganj, the nearest town, 16 km. away or at Bahrampur city, 32 km. away from the village.

Sagardighi Block has one of the major and extensive Integrated Child Development Scheme (ICDS) Projects running in the village of Santoshpur and also in the surrounding villages of the Block. In the study village, ICDS has sponsored several Anganwadi Centres. To make the project more acceptable to the village population, the ICDS project has employed women from the village itself and trained them to run the day-care centres and the crèches. But it has been observed that none of the benefits go to the people they are meant for and are in need, as the women who run these centres and crèches keep most of the food for their own household's consumption, rather than distributing it amongst the pregnant and lactating women and children.

An Integrated Rural Development Programme (IRDP) is also run in the study village and the Block, as well as in the surrounding villages by the government of India for rapid rural development.

Housing condition

The survey data shows that around 91 per cent of the surveyed households had earth flooring and mud walls. More than half of the households (53%) are thatched, and the remaining have roofs either of tiles, tin, or concrete. The main source of drinking water for the village is the public hand pump, and of the surveyed households 84 per cent are dependent on the public hand pump for drinking water. For a majority of the villagers, and an overwhelming 81 per cent of the surveyed households, the pond or the lake is the main source of water for bathing, washing clothes and utensils. Of the 100 households surveyed, 28 per cent had electricity and the remaining used kerosene lamp for lighting. A majority of the households (47%) were using wood and cow-dung cakes as fuel for cooking. Almost 69 per cent of the households cooked their food in a separate cooking place, which more often than not was a corner of the verandah, made into a make-shift kitchen. Most of the houses have one (35%) to four (23%) rooms. Almost 77 per cent of the surveyed population do not have any toilet/latrine facility.

Land holdings and cultivation

Only about one half of the population own agricultural land, and of those who do own some kind of agricultural land, almost half of them depend on rain for irrigation purposes. About fifteen per cent of the farmers and cultivators grow only rice. Another 23 per cent grow wheat, vegetables, mustard, and potatoes as well as rice. As this region of the State is prone to sudden flash floods, most of the farmers have other occupation besides cultivation for subsistence and survival. Most of the agricultural work in the fields is done by family members (34%), and most of what is grown is used for subsistence in a majority of the cases.

More than three quarters (79%) of the households surveyed had some kind of livestock to supplement their income. The cattle and other livestock were generally kept outside the house in cattle-sheds at night and the smaller livestock like the hens, ducks, goats etc. were kept indoors at night.

Assets

Santoshpur village can be compared in economic terms with the village of Kapgari in district Medinipur. In this village as in Kapgari, almost one half of the population surveyed owned either a wrist watch/clock, 17 per cent had electric fans, and a further 37 per cent owned a radio/transistor, and about 11 per cent of the households had a television set. Amongst the surveyed population more than one half of the households owned a bicycle (52%) and only around 13 per cent owned a Bullock/Ox driven cart.

Family type, composition, occupation and income
About one half of the households surveyed were nuclear and the remaining were either joint or joint extended families. In the nuclear families there were three to five children. In the population surveyed, there were 335 males to 289 females (ratio favourable to males). Total population of the survey (all ages) was 624, out of which 252 persons were literate (40%). About 36 per cent, that is, 219 persons had obtained some form of formal education. Normal family size in the village varied between five to seven members in a nuclear family. The most common preferred family composition of the village is of four male children and one female offspring.

An overwhelming 84 per cent of the women surveyed took on the dual roles of being a housewife as well as working with their spouse outside the home. A majority of the women surveyed fetch water, collect wood and dung for fuel, tend to the cattle, look after the elderly and sick, children, cook, clean, and also help out in the fields during harvesting and sowing seasons. They also thresh and winnow grains, prepare puffed rice and rice crisps, for selling and for home consumption. Comparatively, 38 per cent of men run their own small business, 35 per cent work as labourers, and 10 per cent are either employed in public or private sector jobs. Men just work outside the house and do not do anything to help with the household chores. The total monthly income of the surveyed population of the village varied between Rupees 100 to Rupees 2,500, with the mean being in the range of Rs. 501-1000 per month.

Health care utilisation and perception
As the village is situated within the Block headquarters of Sagardighi and the Block Primary Health Centre (BPHC) is just walking distance from the village of Santoshpur, an overwhelming percentage (97%) of women surveyed are aware of the services provided by the BPHC. Interestingly enough, almost all of the households surveyed utilised the services and facilities provided by the BPHC. Despite the dependence on the BPHC for treatment and other purposes, around 72 per cent of the population also consulted with a private doctor or visited a private hospital/clinic for a second opinion.

Although the BPHC is used very frequently for treatment of minor ailments like coughs and colds, influenza, fever and minor cuts and wounds, for major ailments the surveyed population preferred to consult a private physician. More than three quarters of the population surveyed (85%) faced some difficulties and problems in seeking treatment from the BPHC. The most common problem was that medicines were never available at the BPHC. Nonetheless, they still utilised the services of the BPHC for free consultation and prescriptions. More than one half (58%) of the households surveyed thought the BPHC was giving them a 'satisfactory' service, whereas 37 per cent of the population were of the opinion that the health centre was 'fair'. The villagers of Santoshpur make use of the BPHC whenever the need arises, and during emergencies, as it is close to home and the BPHC Doctors are on call 24 hours a day. A majority of the households surveyed feel that the health centre is a blessing for them, as it is easily accessible. But, for treatment of major ailments they prefer to go to the district hospital or consult with a private doctor, since medicines are seldom available at the BPHC.

Medical pluralism is rampant in the village. Of the households surveyed, almost a third of the population try out all sorts of alternative medication before going to the health centre. In case of an illness in the family, the head of the family (normally a male) makes all the decision regarding the type of treatment to be sought by the patient.

It's been found from the survey data that 10 per cent of the males and 9 per cent of the females first try out western medicines at home in case of illness. However, 17 per cent of the males prefer to consult with a private doctor at home as opposed to only 3 per cent of the women surveyed. The women of this village have more faith in homeopathic treatment. Almost a quarter of the women (23%) as compared to 11 per cent of men prefer homeopathy, and in case of an illness, first try this mode of treatment.

About one third of the women (30%) and a quarter of the men (25%) of the survey population prefer "other" types of treatment, normally Shamanistic rituals. It seems that the people of Santoshpur have an immense belief in the existence of supernatural beings. Only about 45 per cent of the males and 43 per cent of the females utilise the services of the BPHC outright without trying other alternative forms of medical practice.

According to a majority of the population surveyed in Santhoshpur, dysentery and diarrhoea is perceived as a major ailment (89%), followed by cholera (54%), tuberculosis (50%) and bronchitis (39%). They classified coughs and colds (78%), headaches (66%) and fevers (60%) as minor ailments. Though they thought these ailments to be minor, they promptly visited the BPHC for consultation and treatment.

Though 18 per cent of the surveyed households thought that influenza was nothing to worry about, although almost three quarters of the population went to the health centre for the treatment of influenza. This can be attributed to the fact that since the BPHC is close to home, the people of Santhoshpur do not hesitate to utilise the facilities and services available even for an ailment which they consider a minor complaint.

Village Sultanpur (District Barddhaman)

Location of the study area

The district of Barddhaman lies to the north-west of Calcutta and is approximately 178 km. from the centre of the city. The study was conducted in a village of this district called Sultanpur, which is administered by the Block headquarters of Memari police station. The village is about 2 km. from the nearest town and is 18 km. from the district city headquarters of Barddhaman. The village is well connected by bus routes and railways. The village is 2 km. from the national and state highway, and the railway station is about 3 km. from the centre of the village. The journey from either the railway station or the bus-stop is normally covered by either bicycles or bullock-carts or by foot. The approach road to the village itself from the highway is an unsurfaced pathway. The district is well connected by railways and roadways. The district headquarters at Barddhaman are connected by rail and road with the state headquarters Calcutta. Both the district headquarters of Barddhaman and the sub-divisional headquarters at Asansol are important industrial towns and railway junctions.

District Barddhaman is predominantly an agricultural district and is appropriately known as the 'granary of West Bengal.' The principal crops grown in this district are rice, cotton, jute, potato, wheat and green vegetables. The district has a very good network of irrigation facilities. The main sources of irrigation are the government canals, tanks, wells and tube-wells. The district is also a major industrial giant in the region and is one of the leading coal mining regions in the state.

Physical setting

The district of Barddhaman is inhabited by all sorts of people from all walks of life. It cannot be said that the district of Barddhaman is predominantly inhabited by a particular religious group, caste group or tribal group. The district was chosen with socio-economic development criteria in mind. Village Sultanpur's surveyed population is composed of 84 per cent Hindu, and 16 per cent Muslim. Of the 84 per cent Hindu population, 4 per cent belong to the Scheduled Tribes, followed by Scheduled Castes (55%), 20 per cent are Kayasthas and the remaining 5 per cent belong to the Brahmin caste.

Sultanpur is about 2 km. from the main road, which is also the national highway connecting the city of Delhi with Calcutta. On the other side of the national highway is the railway station of Memari and the Block headquarters Memari. The railway connects the village and the Block with the district town of Barddhaman, 18 km. away and the city of Calcutta, 181 km. away from the Block headquarters. The village is well linked and served by road and railways and availability and accessibility of transportation are no problem for the villagers of Sultanpur.

The road leading into the village is a beaten and dusty track. On the way to the village is the co-operative store and office, the school and several small ponds. Public hand-pumps are at a distance of every five or six yards from where most of the villagers collect drinking water. At the entrance to the village are the houses of the tribal people, next to this settlement are the houses of the Scheduled Caste people. The more concrete and sturdy houses belong to the upper caste people, who are pretty well off both economically and with regard to social standing.

The Anganwadi Centre is a small structure in the middle of the village. There are no shops within the village. The villagers either have to walk the 2 km. distance or cycle towards the railway station which is the centre of activity. This is where the post office, bank, cinemas, marketplace, grocers and all other shops, chemists and private doctors, both western and traditional, are situated. The village is very peaceful, surrounded by coconut trees, some rice fields and plenty of ponds.

The population
According to the 1981 census, the total land area of Sultanpur is 224.92 hectares, and the total population is 1562 out of which 670 persons are literate (43%). There are 270 households in the village. The PHC is located at the Block headquarters which is 2 km. from the village. Most of the facilities and amenities are available at the Block headquarters. The village has only a few skeletal welfare institutions and social and administrative units. The demographic features are presented in the next page.

According to the 1981 census village Sultanpur's main source of irrigation is by Government Canal (GC), and this source irrigates about 156.21 hectares of land. The area not available for cultivation is 68.71 hectares. The staple diet of this area is also rice and wheat, similar to those of the other districts and villages surveyed. The village has electricity.

Population	Total	Male	Female
	1562	812	750
(i) General	1192	618	574
(ii) Scheduled Castes	285	153	132
(iii) Scheduled Tribes	85	41	44
Economic Activities			
(i) Main Workers	464	400	64
(ii) Cultivators	139	138	01
(iii) Agricultural Labourers	213	158	55
(iv) Household Industry	11	09	02
(v) Other Workers	101	95	06
(vi) Marginal Workers	...	...	...
(vii) Non-Workers	1098	412	686
Literate	670	418	252

Amenities Available	
(i) Educational	P, M, (Grades 1-VI)
(ii) Medical	BPHC (- 2 km.)
(iii) Drinking Water (Potable)	W, TW (Well and Tube-well)
(iv) Post and Telegraph	(- 2 km.) away
(v) Day or Days of the Market, if any	(- 2 km.) away
(vi) Communication BS and Rly. Stn.	(- 2 km.) away
(vii) Approach to Village	PR (Pukka Rd.), & KR (Kuccha Rd.)
(viii) Nearest Town and distance in Km.	Memari 2 km. & Barddhaman 18 km.

(*Source*: District Census Handbook, District Barddhaman, 1981).

Facilities and amenities

The Block headquarters of Memari and the village have almost all the same facilities as the other surveyed villages. This village has the best-run Anganwadi Centre as compared to the other villages studied. The Anganwadi workers are conscientious and regularly visits homes of pregnant and lactating women, keep a close watch on the growth of the infants and children, and provide a referral service. The Anganwadi Centre also distributes iron/folic tablets to pregnant women and administers tetanus injections to the pregnant women. They encourage women to register for antenatal clinics and post natal check-ups along with their infants and keep a record of the immunisation of the new born and accordingly inform parents when the next dose of polio or other vaccination is to be taken from the BPHC for the infants.

The village has a primary, and middle (Grades I-VI) school within the village. All the other facilities are available at the Block Memari which is at a distance of 2 km. from the village. The Block has a Primary Health Centre, also known as the Block Primary Health Centre (BPHC), a Veterinary Hospital, Offices of the 'Gram Panchayat' (also Communist in this village), the Block Development Office (BDO). The premises of the Integrated Child Development Scheme (ICDS), and Integrated Rural Development Project offices are also in Block Memari, adjacent to the Block Development Office (BDO). The post office and the State Bank are close to the national highway and the railway station. The police station is close to the market place. The ration shop, co-operative control shop and the revenue offices are also in the market place of Memari.

Housing condition

The survey data from 100 households show that more than one half of the houses have tiled roofs (55%) followed by a quarter of the houses having concrete roofs (24%), 51 per cent of the houses had concrete walls and 42 per cent mud walls. 61 per cent of the houses had earth floors as opposed to 38 per cent with concrete flooring. The main source of drinking water for half of the surveyed households was the public hand pump. More than one third of the houses (40%) had their own hand pump in the yard/plot/compound of the household and 5 per cent had piped water in their home. About 58 per cent of the population use the ponds for bathing and washing purposes. Of the 100 households surveyed only about one third (30%) had electricity. The rest were dependent on kerosene lamps for lighting.

Of the surveyed households, 40 per cent used coal/lignite as fuel for cooking purposes, followed by a third (33%) who used kerosene and bio-gas as fuel for cooking. Very few (14%) of the households still used firewood as fuel. Almost 40 per cent of the households also had a separate room for cooking, which is generally away from the main house. Most of the houses had one (49%) to two (34%) rooms. Though 60 per cent of the households do not have any toilet/latrine facility, nonetheless, more than one-third of the households (38%) have their own flush toilet/latrine within the compound of the house.

Land holdings and cultivation

A mere seven per cent of the surveyed households owned any agricultural land. Most of the land owned by the farmers was irrigated by government canals. Of those who owned some kind of land, almost everybody grew only rice and all their family members helped with the work in the fields. For most of them the income generated by the land is enough for their subsistence. About 40 per cent of the households had some kind of livestock and most of them kept the cattle outside the main house, in cattle-sheds in the household compound at night. Small livestock were kept indoors at night.

Assets

The village of Sultanpur is comparable to the other study villages of Kapgari and Santhoshpur in terms of economic status of the population surveyed. In this village too, more than one half of the households (52%) owned a radio/transistor, 49 per cent possessed a clock/wrist watch. Only about 17 per cent had electric fans, 16 per cent owned a television set, 6 per cent had sofa sets, followed by a minuscule percentage owning refrigerators, a car, a motorcycle/scooter etc. The percentage owning bicycles was comparatively lower than in the other villages. Only about 40 percent of the population surveyed had a bicycle, and no one had a bullock/ox driven cart. This may be due to the close proximity to the district town and easy accessibility of all kinds and means of transportation to almost all the major places of the district and to the city of Calcutta.

Family type, composition, occupation and income

Almost all the households surveyed are nuclear, with a family size of four-five members in a nuclear family. A nuclear family had on an average two to three children. The most commonly preferred family size in the village is one female and one male child. In the population surveyed, that is, of 100 households, there were 226 males as opposed to 239 females (the only surveyed village where the ratio is favourable to females). The total population size of the survey was 465, out of which 310 persons were literate (67%), and 259 persons had the opportunity of a formal school education (56%).

More than one half of the surveyed women (58%) are housewives and are responsible for all the household chores and duties of cooking, cleaning, washing, bearing and rearing children. Out of the remaining, a quarter of the women (25%) worked as labourers besides doing the household chores and duties. A further 5 per cent of the women worked in government offices and schools as teachers and clerks. The rest of the women either worked in the fields, or worked as maid servants, or had their own small scale business to run, in addition to household work.

As compared to the women in the survey, a third of the men (30%) were employed in either public or private sector blue collar jobs. A similar percentage of men also worked as labourers, whereas 11 per cent have their own business. The total monthly income of the surveyed households of the village was greater than the other three villages studied so far. The monthly income falls in the range of Rs. 1001-2500 for about 54 per cent of the population.

Health care utilisation and perception

A majority of the women surveyed are aware of the services provided by the Block Primary Health Centre (BPHC) in their Block and village. But, surprisingly, only a very low 7 per cent of the population had ever used the services and facilities of the BPHC. Nearly 90 per cent of the population surveyed preferred the district government hospital over the BPHC, or else preferred to consult with a private doctor (62%).

Of those who ever used the BPHC, 65 per cent used it for treating minor ailments like coughs and colds, followed by fevers (57%), and 39 per cent also used it for treating dysentery and diarrhoea. Only 12 per cent had encountered any problem or difficulty in seeking treatment from the health centre. The most common complaint was that of 'long waiting time', and some felt that the behaviour of the health staff was rude and discourteous, whereas others complained regarding the poor quality of service. However, 45 per cent of the households commented that the service of the health centre was 'extremely good', followed by 'satisfactory' (42%).

The surveyed households utilise the services of the BPHC in case of an emergency or when all the other avenues are closed. Normally they prefer to take the patient to the district hospital or consult with a private doctor. It has been found that a majority of the people (84% males and 85% females) are directly taken to the district hospital for treatment in case of an illness however major or minor the ailment may be. Before visiting the government hospital, 7 per cent of the women try homeopathy, 2 per cent try home remedies, and a further 2 per cent administer western medicine at home. About 67 per cent of the males and 58 per cent of the females consult a private practitioner at home. Dysentery and diarrhoea are perceived by 68 per cent of the households to be a major ailment. Coughs, colds (85%), fevers (76%) are perceived as minor ailments.

The utilisation of the BPHC is minimal in this village. This is because a majority of the people are economically better off and consider consultation with a private physician more worthwhile than waiting in long queues at the BPHC. Besides, due to the easy accessibility and availability of transportation, proximity to the district town, makes them more mobile and opens up an array of choices.

The following section presents the general health situation of the country and West Bengal state.

Health Situation of India and West Bengal

This section outlines the general health situation of the entire country and the state of West Bengal in comparison to the other major states of India. It also examines the major social indicators such as fertility and mortality within the country by rural/urban residence, life expectancy, and presents distribution of births by type of medical attention received by the mother at delivery.

Mortality Situation in India

One of the striking demographic features in India over the last three-quarters of this century has been the decline in mortality. An examination of the health situation shows that until the first quarter of the present century the mortality was very high. In the early twenties, it was about 45 per thousand but started declining after 1921, and recently dropped to about 9.8 per thousand. The fall in mortality rates in this period can be largely attributed to the control of epidemics which was mainly achieved due to the introduction of massive health programmes and public health measures thereby bringing down the intensity of epidemics and communicable killer diseases like the plague, cholera, smallpox, and malaria.

Improvement in communication and transportation, too, curtailed the death rates further. The decline in the death rate was slow in the beginning, but has been more rapid during the last three decades. Though the death rates declined rapidly it was not uniform within the country (as can be noted from table 3.1).

Wide variation in the levels of death rates between states and by rural-urban residence is observed, despite the services offered through the network of primary health centres (PHC) and sub-centres throughout the country. Improvement in the mortality situation is also reflected in the rising expectation of life at birth. Over the last 75 years, expectation of life at birth has more than doubled, and the average expectation of life is now more than 55 years. Refer to table 3.1, for information on crude death rates, infant mortality rates, and expectation of life at birth within the country.

Infant and Early Childhood Mortality

In comparison with the decline in the general death rate, the fall in the infant

Table 3.1:   **Crude death rates, infant mortality rates (1991), and expectation of life at birth (1990) in India by major states, residence, and sex**

Major States	Crude death rate (CDR)			Infant mortality rate (IMR)			Expectation of Life at Birth		
	Total	Rural	Urban	Total	Rural	Urban	Persons	Males	Females
INDIA	9.8	10.6	7.1	80	87	53	59	58.10	59.10
Andhra Pradesh	9.7	10.5	6.7	73	77	56	-	59.10	62.23
Assam	11.5	11.8	6.9	81	83	42	-	55.74	55.23
Bihar	9.8	10.2	6.3	69	71	46	-	58.21	57.00
Gujarat	8.5	8.8	7.9	69	73	57	-	58.34	61.49
Haryana	8.2	8.5	6.8	68	73	49	-	63.41	61.97
Himachal Pradesh	8.9	9.1	5.2	75	76	38	-	-	-
Karnataka	9.0	9.8	6.9	77	87	47	-	62.15	63.31
Kerala	6.0	6.2	5.3	16	17	16	-	66.23	71.12
Madhya Pradesh	13.8	14.9	9.2	117	125	74	-	56.24	54.71
Maharashtra	8.2	9.3	6.2	60	69	38	-	61.90	62.91
Orissa	12.8	13.5	6.5	124	129	71	-	57.13	55.15
Punjab	7.8	8.5	5.7	53	58	40	-	65.61	65.30
Rajasthan	10.1	10.6	7.7	79	84	50	-	57.80	58.69
Tamil Nadu	8.8	9.5	7.6	57	65	42	-	60.85	60.80
Uttar Pradesh	11.3	12.0	8.3	97	102	74	-	54.14	49.64
West Bengal	8.3	8.9	6.7	71	76	47	-	59.95	59.53

• excludes Jammu and Kashmir

(*Source:* Sample Registration System: Fertility and Mortality Indicators, 1991; State of the World's Children, UNICEF, 1992; and Family Welfare Yearbook, 1989-90)

mortality rate has been much slower. The infant mortality rate is an excellent summary index of the level of living and socio-economic development of a country and is a sensitive index of health conditions prevailing in a society. The infant mortality rates of the major states of India are presented in table 3.1. The reduction in infant mortality to a large extent depends on the availability of medical facilities to the expectant mothers in the rural areas in the antenatal period; the extent of births attended by trained medical practitioners at the medical institutions; the care of the infant and child soon after birth, and the associated social and economic circumstances of the household. However, a large proportion of births in the rural areas take place at home and are not attended by any trained medical practitioners. The type of medical attention received at birth is an important factor influencing the level of infant morbidity and mortality. Infant deaths constitute nearly 30 per cent of total deaths within the country (Padmanabha, 1985).

Infant mortality in the rural areas has always been higher than in the urban areas and has remained so over the years. This reflects either the lack of proper medical facilities in the rural areas or the absence of services in the antenatal period, and under-utilisation of maternal and child health care services. These factors appear to contribute to the higher levels of mortality in the rural areas among infants. More than one half of the births are attended by untrained professionals and others in the rural areas, as opposed to 19 per cent in the urban areas. Table 3.2 presents the births attended by trained and untrained practitioners in the rural and urban areas of India and the major states.

Table 3.2:   **Per cent distribution of births by type of medical attention received by the mother at delivery by residence, India and major states, (1991)**

Major States	Institutional			Attended by Trained Professionals			Attended by Untrained Professionals and others		
	Total	Rural	Urban	Total	Rural	Urban	Total	Rural	Urban
INDIA*	24.3	17.6	53.8	21.9	20.8	26.9	53.7	61.5	19.2
Andhra Pradesh	37.7	21.4	78.1	19.6	24.5	7.5	42.7	54.2	14.4
Assam	18.3	12.9	50.9	10.7	9.8	16.2	71.0	77.3	32.9
Bihar	11.7	9.5	28.2	15.3	13.5	29.2	72.9	76.9	42.6
Gujarat	23.5	16.3	64.8	33.6	36.6	16.2	42.9	47.1	19.0
Haryana	19.9	16.9	32.7	64.5	65.4	60.9	15.6	17.7	6.5
Himachal Pradesh	21.5	16.4	49.1	23.8	20.3	42.8	54.8	63.3	8.1
Karnataka	40.6	30.5	73.4	23.5	26.2	14.8	35.9	43.3	11.9
Kerala	91.5	90.6	95.3	5.0	5.3	3.7	3.6	4.1	1.0
Madhya Pradesh	13.2	5.3	50.2	14.1	13.0	19.1	72.8	81.7	30.8
Maharashtra	34.3	20.9	75.9	15.5	14.8	17.7	50.2	64.2	6.4
Orissa	9.8	6.4	33.8	18.0	16.6	27.8	75.2	80.5	38.5
Punjab	7.3	5.2	13.0	87.2	87.9	85.2	5.5	7.0	1.8
Rajasthan	5.0	2.6	16.8	19.4	16.7	33.0	75.7	80.6	50.2
Tamil Nadu	56.8	46.2	89.1	18.8	22.7	6.8	24.2	31.1	4.1
Uttar Pradesh	4.5	2.7	14.1	26.6	20.1	61.1	68.8	77.1	24.8
West Bengal	30.7	23.4	78.0	9.3	9.0	11.5	60.0	67.6	10.5

•   excludes Jammu and Kashmir

(*Source*: Sample Registration System: Fertility and Mortality Indicators, 1991)

Another factor which has an influence on the level of infant mortality is the type of medical attention received before death. Among infants, the major cause of death in most parts of the rural areas of the country is tetanus. In the rural areas as well as in the urban areas, tetanus, pneumonia and dysentery, along with typhoid, account for high proportions of deaths among children aged between one to three years. In addition, influenza also is responsible for a high proportion of deaths among children (Padmanabha, 1985).

According to the 1979 Survey on Infant and Child Mortality in India, the major and 'most frequent' causes of death in the country are tetanus, followed by dysentery and diarrhoea. Prematurity and various other respiratory ailments like pneumonia, bronchitis and influenza are the other major causes influencing infant mortality.

Earlier studies suggest that antenatal care can lead to a significant decline in the neonatal mortality rate. Some of the important factors which cause high neonatal mortality in India and particularly in the rural areas, are the place of delivery, type of attendant at childbirth and the practices followed with respect to care of the new-born (Visaria, 1985). Female mortality among infants in India, is generally higher than male infants, especially in the rural areas. The sex differentials in morbidity and mortality of infants and children show that in parts of the country a lower value is given to the girls than to the boys. Table 3.3 presents the infant mortality rates by sex and residence.

Maternal Mortality

According to UNICEF (1990), the Maternal Mortality Rate (MMR), of India was 460 per 100,000 births. Higher mortality for females in India is a reflection of the role and status of women, both within the family and in society at large, and represents the health consequences of social, economic and cultural discrimination against them. The health status of women has a two-fold significance. First women constitute almost half of the population and their condition contributes to the overall health situation and second, women's health determines the health of the future population (Karkal, 1987). The causes of maternal deaths are haemorrhage, infection, and pregnancy-induced hypertension (toxaemia or eclampsia) often with anaemia, and sepsis. Despite unnecessary suffering and deaths caused by lack of appropriate care during pregnancy and childbirth, only about 22 per cent of the births in India are assisted by trained attendants, and 24 per cent of the births are institutionalised (refer to table 3.2 for more information).

Table 3.3:   **Estimated infant mortality rates by sex and residence, India, and major states, (1991)**

Major States	Combined			Rural			Urban		
	Person	Male	Female	Person	Male	Female	Person	Male	Female
INDIA*	80	81	80	87	87	87	53	53	52
Andhra Pradesh	73	76	70	77	78	75	56	65	47
Assam	81	88	74	83	90	76	42	49	36
Bihar	69	68	71	71	70	73	46	46	45
Gujarat	69	70	67	73	76	70	57	56	58
Haryana	68	69	67	73	74	71	49	48	51
Himachal Pradesh	75	81	67	76	82	69	38	49	27
Karnataka	77	82	72	87	91	82	47	51	43
Kerala	16	17	16	17	17	16	16	17	15
Madhya Pradesh	117	116	119	125	123	127	74	75	73
Maharashtra	60	60	59	69	69	70	38	42	33
Orissa	124	126	123	129	131	127	71	72	69
Punjab	53	55	51	58	60	56	40	41	38
Rajasthan	79	77	80	84	83	85	50	47	54
Tamil Nadu	57	60	54	65	69	61	42	43	40
Uttar Pradesh	97	95	100	102	99	105	74	70	77
West Bengal	71	72	69	76	79	73	47	44	49

• excludes Jammu and Kashmir

(*Source*: Sample Registration System: Fertility and Mortality Indicators, 1991)

Malnutrition, including anaemia, is a serious health problem, especially in women who have too many pregnancies too closely spaced and this contributes significantly to maternal morbidity and mortality in developing countries. Too many or too closely spaced pregnancies give rise to health risks both for the mothers and the infants and higher maternal and infant mortality rates. Age at childbearing is another important factor contributing towards maternal mortality. Thus, the neglect and under-nourishment of girls sets in motion a vicious cycle of deteriorating health of the population, and continuing high mortality and morbidity among infants and children.

Health Situation of West Bengal

Compared to the other major states in the country, the overall health situation of West Bengal is not alarming. However, expectation of life at birth is lower than some of the other states, but, higher than the national level. Interestingly enough the crude death rate is lower than both the national level and of the other states, except Punjab, Kerala and Haryana. Nonetheless, infant mortality is higher than some of the other states reflecting either under utilisation of maternal and child health services or lack of available MCH facilities in the state (Refer to table 3.1 and 3.2 for more information and details).

The following tables presents the health situation of the state by outlining the health personnel working in the rural areas, hospitals, dispensaries and beds available and average population served, number of doctors and average population served, deaths due to diarroheal diseases, tetanus, malaria, tuberculosis, etc., and deaths related to childbirth and pregnancy, in the state of West Bengal. Table 3.4, shows the overall distribution of doctors engaged by a government agency, such as the central and state government hospitals, public sector undertaking hospital, etc., and the population served per doctor in the major states of the country. West Bengal's ratio of population served per doctor is comparatively better than most other states of India (Refer to table 3.4 for more information). The table shows that West Bengal ranked fourth in 1989, within the country with regards to average population served per doctor.

Table 3.4:   **Number of doctors and average population served in major states (1989)**

Major States	Doctors Engaged Under (Government Agency)	Total	Population Served per Doctor
Andhra Pradesh	+	32227*	1: 1960
Assam	2660	2660	1: 8783
Bihar	+	24486	1: 3387
Gujarat	2835	2835	1: 14015
Haryana	1289	1289	1: 12282
Himachal Pradesh	916	916	1: 5400
Karnataka	+	29501*	1: 1511
Kerala	4163	4163	1: 7126
Madhya Pradesh	+	9060	1: 6825
Maharashtra	+	62770*	1: 1182
Orissa	5045	5045	1: 6027
Punjab	3462	3462	1:5653
Rajasthan	+	12243*	1: 3461
Tamil Nadu	8207	8207	1: 6784
Uttar Pradesh	8377	8377	1: 1563
West Bengal	+	30092	1: 2154

•   excludes Jammu and Kashmir

(*Source*: Health Information India - 1990)

Note: * = Registered Number of Doctors; + = Not Available
        Government Agency includes Central/State Government Hospital, Public Sector Undertaking Hospital Etc. (Figures Are Provisional)

Tables 3.5, 3.6, 3.7, display the distribution of health personnel (medical specialists, medical doctors, and paramedical staff) working in the rural areas of West Bengal (Refer to the tables).

Table 3.5:   **Health manpower working in rural West Bengal (1990); medical specialists working at upgraded PHCs/CHCs**

SL. NO.	SURGEONS		OBST. & GYNAES		PHYSICIANS		PAEDIATRICIANS		TOTAL SPECIALISTS	
	S	P	S	P	S	P	S	P	S	P
India	672	455	620	356	613	490	522	285	3053	2228
Andhra Pradesh	Nil	Nil	Nil	Nil	Nil	Nil	Nil	Nil	Nil	Nil
Assam	8	4	8	6	8*	2*	INR	INR	24	12
Bihar	INR	INR	INR	INR	INR	INR	INR	INR	INR	INR
Gujarat	159	88	63	39	24	18	63	20	309	165
Haryana	21	6	21	5	21	3	21	2	114	83
Himachal Pradesh	15	15	6	6	15	15	6	6	42	42
Karnataka	62	61	24	23	59	57	20	17	165	158
Kerala	INR	INR	INR	INR	87	87	INR	INR	87	87
Madhya Pradesh	86	49	97	56	86	52	97	42	366	199
Maharashtra	INR	INR	INR	INR	INR	INR	INR	INR	161	160
Orissa	0	Nil	66	66	Nil	Nil	66	52	132	118
Punjab	46	43	46	43	46uc	43uc	INR	INR	138	129
Rajasthan	INR	INR	INR	INR	INR	INR	INR	INR	425	415
Tamil Nadu	30	30	30	30	147	147	Nil	Nil	207	207
Uttar Pradesh	142	96	144	26	6	4	142	123	434	249
West Bengal	70	42	80	41	80	39	80	11	320	133

•   excludes Jammu and Kashmir

(*Source*: Health Information India - 1990)

Note: S = Number Sanctioned;   P = Number in Position
INR = Information Not Received;   uc = Under Clarification
* = Including Paediatricians, As Separate Figures Not Available
(Figures are Provisional)

Table 3.6:   **Health manpower employed in**
rural areas (1990)
medical doctors at PHCs

SL. NO.	Doctors at PHCs	
	S (No. Sanctioned)	P (No. in Position)
India	24332	20248
Andhra Pradesh	1916	1555
Assam	584	584
Bihar	2121	2121
Gujarat	774	616
Haryana	645	433
Himachal Pradesh	264	249
Karnataka	945@@	816@@
Kerala	1087	1087
Madhya Pradesh	1647	1347
Maharashtra	3422	2947
Orissa	942	548
Punjab	1706	1615
Rajasthan	961	953
Tamil Nadu	1369	1251
Uttar Pradesh	3787	2263
West Bengal	1413	1203

● excludes Jammu and Kashmir

(*Source*: Health Information India - 1990)

Note: @@ = Revised Figure Received From Karnataka State.
(Figures Are Provisional)

Table 3.7:   **Health manpower working in rural areas**
of India and West Bengal, paramedical
(1990)

Health Manpower (Paramedical)	INDIA		WEST BENGAL	
	S	P	S	P
Block Extension Educators	6117	5594	341	317
Health Assistants (Male)	26658	24549	1689	1689
Health Assistants (Female)/LHVs	21710	17717	1689	947
Health Workers (Male)	89142	82122	10134	9120
Health Workers (Female)/ANM	132225	120572	10134	8126
Pharmacists	21683	19733	1252	1163
Laboratory Technicians	10406	8801	439	374
Nurse-Midwives	16447	13880	3544	3004

(*Source*: Health Information India - 1990)

Note: (Figures Are Provisional)

The following tables 3.8 and 3.9 represent the distribution and numbers of hospitals and dispensaries, available beds and population served according to rural urban areas in India and the major states (Refer to the tables). The tables show that most of the hospitals are concentrated in the urban centres.

Table 3.8:   **Number of hospitals, beds and population served according to rural/urban areas (1990)**

SL. NO.	Rural		Urban		Total		Population Served Per Bed
	Hospitals	Beds	Hospitals	Beds	Hospitals	Beds	
India	3167	95722	7005	506768	10172	602490	1364
Andhra Pradesh ('86)	165	3716	450	32684	615	36400	1905
Assam ('89)	107	3362	96	10895	203	14257	1677
Bihar ('88)	76	2298	222	25839	298	28137	2884
Gujarat ('89)	130	5010	1433	41364	1563	46374	857
Haryana	8	543	69	6900	77	7443	2168
Himachal Pradesh	23	598	42	3716	65	4314	1165
Karnataka	25	2526	261	31442	286	33968	1312
Kerala	1631	41033	422	32651	2053	73684	403
Madhya Pradesh ('89)	83	1967	279	20136	362	22103	2798
Maharashtra ('88)	222	9066	1659	83909	1881	92975	775
Orissa	121	2539	166	11049	287	13588	2276
Punjab ('89)	116	3549	149	12545	265	16094	1201
Rajasthan	27	1376	239	19784	266	21160	2055
Tamil Nadu	89	4235	319	44545	408	48780	1141
Uttar Pradesh ('86)	83	2585	652	44693	735	47278	2577
West Bengal	131	7610	279	46367	410	53977	1201

• excludes Jammu and Kashmir

(*Source*: Health Information India - 1990)

Table 3.9:   **Number of dispensaries and beds according to rural/urban areas (1990)**

SL. NO.	Rural		Urban		Total	
	Dispensaries	Beds	Dispensaries	Beds	Dispensaries	Beds
India	12747	13642	15557	9286	28304	22928
Andhra Pradesh ('86)	549	171	244	106	793	277
Assam ('89)	300	6	18	42	318	48
Bihar ('88)	411	-	16	96	427	96
Gujarat ('89)	2470	637	3388	4013	5858	4650
Haryana	39	29	175	373	214	402
Himachal Pradesh	187	184	22	27	209	211
Karnataka	818	581	215	270	1033	851
Kerala	1240	61	508	44	1748	105
Madhya Pradesh ('89)	278	132	87	83	365	215
Maharashtra ('88)	842	403	8293	1948	9135	2351
Orissa	134	75	64	4	198	79
Punjab ('89)	1341	5342	226	648	1567	5990
Rajasthan	546	376	418	807	964	1183
Tamil Nadu	147	138	365	140	512	278
Uttar Pradesh ('86)	1318	5137	432	592	1750	5729
West Bengal	408	-	143	-	551	-

• excludes Jammu and Kashmir

(*Source:* Health Information India - 1990)

Note: - = Nil Information

The following tables. 3.10 and 3.11, describes the reported cases and deaths due to diarrhoeal diseases, meningitis, malaria, tetanus, whooping cough, measles and tuberculosis in India and in some of the major states (Refer to the tables).

Table 3.10:   **Reported cases and deaths due to diarrhoeal diseases, meningitis, and malaria in India by major states (1989)**

Major States	Cholera @		Acute Diarrhoeal Diseases		Meningitis		Malaria	
	Cases (C)	Deaths (D)	Cases (C)	Deaths (D)	Cases	Deaths	Cases	Deaths
INDIA	5044	72	9288242	4791	19619	2644	2017823	268
Andhra Pradesh	201	-	1177934	627	1313*	80	82510	2
Assam	-	-	723889	238	-*	-	62274	6
Bihar	-	-	21412	26	1014	42	40001	13
Gujarat	275	5	240190	393	2329	524	598653	60
Haryana	4	-	272947	149	6*	1	23711	-
Himachal Pradesh	-	-	478731	97	72*	8	8589	-
Karnataka	770	26	265833	179	-*	-	106683	-
Kerala	139	7	733826	141	325*	7	6126	1
Madhya Pradesh	35	1	1046693	621	440#*	481	252886	16
Maharashtra	56	2	435455	314	3090	674	122314	8
Orissa	-	-	1352123	958	4249*	404	260815	118
Punjab	5	-	181815	86	17*	3	32146	2
Rajasthan	1	-	106790	36	585#*	75	112316	1
Tamil Nadu	3231	30	54992	124	19*	3	90478	-
Uttar Pradesh	91	-	626088	291	4*	-	101815	-
West Bengal	37	-	+	+	+*	+	18822	16

•   excludes Jammu and Kashmir

(*Source:* Health Information India - 1990)

Note: - = Nil;   + = Not Available
@ = Notified Cases of Cholera based on Weekly Epidemiological Reports
# = Brain Fever;   * = Meningococcal Meningitis

Table 3.11:   **Reported cases and deaths due to tetanus, whooping cough, measles and tuberculosis in India and major states (1989)**

Major States	Tetanus		Whooping Cough		Measles		Tuberculosis	
	C	D	C	D	C	D	C	D
INDIA	16674	2007	146046	69	157247	664	1040772	9382
Andhra Pradesh	1763	243	22624	11	21815	59	209870	1206
Assam	281	90	11429	7	9886	3	32849	122
Bihar	133	12	6416	4	1340	-	5377	37
Gujarat	536	115	4406	21	6356	227	36306	442
Haryana	450	63	513	-	651	-	40154	407
Himachal Pradesh	53	9	567	-	4446	4	19463	366
Karnataka	2789	157	3566	-	8706	20	82139	944
Kerala	90	7	6605	3	26187	6	62139	281
Madhya Pradesh	1913	182	30594	8	12086	35	89272	291
Maharashtra	1325	323	504	3	8648	46	93032	1305
Orissa	2769	281	23772	1	13197	15	69960	802
Punjab	123	46	1623	2	551	9	12512	123
Rajasthan	371	42	1190	1	2492	17	61174	352
Tamil Nadu	107	13	1063	3	11068	111	25486	250
Uttar Pradesh	1772	247	17477	-	7301	17	46603	198
West Bengal	+	+	+	+	+	+	+	+

•   excludes Jammu and Kashmir

(*Source:* Health Information India - 1990)

Note: C = Cases;   D = Deaths;   - = Nil
        + = Not Available

   Table 3.12 presents the percentage distribution of diseases and infantile illness leading to death in India between 1982-1987.

Table 3.12:   **Percentage distribution of specific causes of death under the group of diseases peculiar to infancy - India, 1982-1987**

Causes	1982	1983	1984	1985	1986	1987
Prematurity	37.3	43.6	45.3	41.4	41.0	43.9
Malposition	1.0	0.1	-	-	-	-
Congenital Malformation	1.5	2.4	2.6	-	2.6	2.3
Birth Injury	2.1	2.5	1.9	2.2	2.5	2.0
Respiratory Infection of New Born	12.1	13.7	15.5	13.5	14.5	16.6
Cord Infection	2.6	8.1	5.8	6.8	7.7	6.9
Diahorrea of New Born	10.4	9.5	8.9	11.3	10.2	10.0
Malnutrition	10.3	1.8	-	-	-	-
Convulsion	7.0	0.7	-	-	-	-
Not Classifiable	15.7	17.6	20.6	24.8	21.5	18.3

(*Source*: Health Information India - 1990)

Note: - = Nil

Table 3.13 and 3.14 presents deaths of mothers related to childbirth and pregnancy.

Table 3.13:   **Percentage distribution of deaths by causes related to childbirth and pregnancy (maternal) 1982-1987**

Specific Causes	1982	1983	1984	1985	1986	1987
Abortion	10.1	10.7	10.8	11.5	8.0	7.6
Toxaemia	12.5	12.1	10.8	6.7	11.9	6.6
Anaemia	24.4	18.9	23.3	23.1	17.0	17.8
Bleeding in Pregnancy and Puerperium	26.2	23.8	18.8	15.9	21.6	27.9
Malposition of Child leading to Death of Mother	7.2	8.3	6.2	7.7	6.2	10.1
Puerperium Sepsis	8.3	11.6	10.8	13.9	13.1	10.7
Non Classifiable Symptoms	11.3	14.6	19.3	21.2	22.2	19.3
Per cent of Total Deaths	1.2	1.2	1.0	1.2	1.0	1.0

(*Source*: Survey of Causes of Deaths (Rural) Annual Report 1986, Registrar General, India)

Table 3.14:   **Percentage distribution of deaths by causes related to childbirth and pregnancy (maternal mortality) in India - 1987**

Specific Causes		Age Group in Years		
	Total Deaths (%)	15-24 (%)	25-34 (%)	35-44 (%)
Abortion	7.6	8.6	7.6	5.7
Toxaemia	6.6	8.6	6.5	2.9
Anaemia	17.8	15.7	12.0	37.1
Bleeding in Pregnancy and Puerperium	27.9	34.3	28.3	14.3
Malposition of Child leading to Death of Mother	10.1	10.0	7.6	17.1
Puerperium Sepsis	10.7	7.1	1401	8.6
Non Classifiable Symptoms	19.3	15.7	23.9	14.3

The above tables attempt to present at least a partial picture of the health situation and socio-economic condition of the country and individual states. General social indicators, such as infant and maternal mortality rates provide an excellent summary index for measuring the development of a country and providing comparative data for the state of West Bengal.

Conclusion

The study villages display certain similarities and dissimilarities in their characteristics with regards to population composition, religion, communication and socio-economic development. The data suggests homogeneity and disparity in health care behaviour between the villages. Culture, religion and tradition, have an impact on certain aspects of health care utilisation and behaviour. Furthermore, the study observed the services of the primary health care centres to have limited impact. Medical pluralism was much in evidence in the villages and more than one medical system was used simultaneously depending on the perceived severity of illness.

The study found that with higher socio-economic status health care behaviour changes and utilisation of available health care services also increases, irrespective of religious beliefs, caste or tribal alliance. The ideal family size and composition also changes with higher socio-economic status. However, perceptions about major and minor ailments were found to be very similar in all the study villages irrespective of the educational standards of women and socio-economic status.

India adopted the National Health Policy (NHP) in June 1981 which was approved by the Parliament in 1983. The delivery of health services is mainly governed by the National Health Policy which places a major emphasis on ensuring primary health care to all by the year 2000. As health is seen as a state subject under the Indian Constitution, the responsibility for providing health services are with the State Department of Health and Family Welfare of each state (Kannan et al., 1991). In almost all the states, all the districts have District Hospitals where curative services are provided. The Primary Health Centre (PHC) is the core institution of the rural health services infrastructure in India. As of March 1992, there were 20,719 PHCs and 131,464 sub-centres, providing health and family welfare services to the rural population (Government of India, 1994). The rural health system at present offers family welfare services, including maternal and child health schemes. Furthermore, the National Child Survival and Safe Motherhood (CSSM) Programme provides a package of services combining immunisation with maternal and child health care interventions (Ministry of Health and Family Welfare, 1992).

The National Health Policy recognises the failure of the existing health system to reach women, especially in the rural areas, but still does not specifically discuss women's health issues, nor recognises the importance of improving women's health. Problems of implementation have hampered the effectiveness of the pyramidal health structure and policy which has been established both in the rural and the urban areas. Hence, the NHP's aims to rectify the problem via extensive primary health care approach, with special attention to maternal and child health services, nutrition and immunisation programmes has not been very successful at the grassroots level.

Social Context of Women's Health in Rural India

Sulekha is 26 years old and has three children, two girls and a boy. She was married when she was 15 years old, immediately after attaining puberty. Her husband was then 24 years old. She attended school till the 3rd grade and is able to sign her name and can barely read and write. She dropped out of school because her older brother got married and he wanted Sulekha to live with him and his wife to help out with the household chores. He migrated to another district and Sulekha went with them as a domestic help.

Her husband completed higher secondary education (grade 12) and can read and write competently. He runs his own small scale business earning about Rupees 30-50 a day. Sulekha says that the income they have is enough for the family's subsistence. They have their house, which is made of mud and the roof is tiled, the floors are also made of mud. They have a big living room and a bedroom and a kitchen. They have a tubewell in their yard, so they do not have any water problem. However, they do not have any latrine facility and use the fields or the wooded areas as a latrine.

She had her first child when she was around 17 years old. The next child was born when she was about 19 years old. After that she became pregnant immediately, so she decided to have an induced abortion, with the permission of her husband. She and her husband decided to abort that pregnancy on the advise of their health worker. She went to a private western medical practitioner for an abortion and did not use the facility of the government hospital or the block PHC because they were afraid that the health personnel would not take care of her efficiently and properly as the services were free. After the abortion the doctor advised her against immediate pregnancy and also advised her not to have a child for another four to five years. After that she was on the pill for quite some time. She opted for the reversible contraception because she desperately wanted to have a son. Finally she had a son just prior to the survey. Both she and her husband had vowed to a particular goddess that if they were blessed with a son they would perform certain kind of rituals and offer prayers when their son is six months old.

Some of the demographic characteristics like age, age at first marriage, marital status and so on are discussed here.

Information on age is normally collected by asking the date of birth of the individual (day, month, year) or by asking a direct question to obtain information on age at the last birth day, or by asking both these questions together. Though the question about the date of birth obviously yields more concrete information, it is not always possible to obtain the date of birth from a population in which the majority are either illiterate or semi-literate. In such a situation, information on age is collected by asking about important events they remember like floods, famines, droughts; and in the case of women, when they attained puberty, and so on.

Though it is easy enough to ask questions on age, it is extremely difficult to obtain correct information about age when people are ignorant about their own age. In India, it is not uncommon for investigators or enumerators to be told, 'I do not know my age. Maybe I am 20 or 25 years old. Why don't you decide how old I am?' The practice of registering births is not yet widely followed and therefore, birth certificates are not available. The extent of non-reporting of vital events is found to be very high in the rural areas. One of the basic reasons for this is mass illiteracy and the rural character of the population. For most Indian people, few occasions arise when birth or death certificates are required.

Hence, it was not surprising that I encountered difficulty in enumerating the age of the study population. A majority of the women were ignorant about both their date of birth and their age. Therefore the age structure presented here of the women may not be exactly accurate, as it was obtained after a long discussion of 'the important events' of their lives. A majority of the women were in the reproductive age group of 15-49 years of age, as this (reproductive age group) was the basic requirement of the study. Refer to table 4.1 for the age structure and age-groups of the study population, particularly women.

Table 4.1:   **Age-structure of the study population (Females)**

AGE OF ELIGIBLE WOMEN	MOTIPUR (Tribal)	KAPGARI (Hindu)	SANTOSHPUR (Muslim)	SULTANPUR (Developed)	TOTAL
13-14	-	-	2	-	2 (0.49%)
15-19	8	12	13	10	43 (10.72%)
20-24	19	28	31	15	93 (23.19%)
25-29	36	20	18	34	108 (26.93%)
30-34	16	20	24	19	79 (19.70%)
35-39	11	11	7	19	48 (11.97%)
40-44	12	7	4	3	26 (6.48%)
45-49	-	2	-	-	2 (0.49%)
TOTAL	102	100	99	100	401

The table shows that the highest number of eligible women were in the 25-29 years of age group (nearly one third), closely followed by the 20-24 years age group (almost a quarter). This is because almost all the rural women are married before they reach their twenties owing to the various socio-cultural norms, customs and economic factors associated with marriage.

Age and sex are the basic characteristics of any group and affect its social, economic, political and demographic structure. They are also an important indicator of the social status of people because each individual is ascribed a certain status in society on the basis of their sex and age. Similarly, his/her expected role in the family and society is associated with sex and age. These are culturally determined and vary from one culture to another. It is well known, for instance, that in the traditional Hindu family, men are more important than women and older persons are more important than younger ones.

Almost all the women were currently married at the time of survey. Very few women were either separated, widowed or divorced. An overwhelming 93 per cent of the women in Motipur were currently married, two were separated, and five women were widowed. However, all the women in villages Kapgari and Sultanpur were currently married at the time of the survey. Ninety-five per cent of the women in Santoshpur were currently married, two were divorced, two were widowed and one was separated from her husband.

Almost all the currently married women lived with their husbands. Only in very few cases was this not so, usually when the husbands were away from their village and wives because of their jobs or business or for military service. An overwhelming majority of the women were very young at the time of their first marriage. Refer to table 4.2, for more details of age at marriage.

Table 4.2:   Age of women at the time of first marriage (Percentage)

AGE AT THE TIME OF CURRENT MARRIAGE	MOTIPUR (Tribal)	KAPGARI (Hindu)	SANTOSHPUR (Muslim)	SULTANPUR (Developed)	TOTAL
8-14	23	30	51	24	128 (31.92%)
15-19	45	41	44	62	192 (47.88%)
20-24	12	14	4	12	42 (10.47%)
25 +	1	2	-	2	5 (1.24%)
DON'T KNOW	21	13	-	-	34 (8.47%)
TOTAL	102	100	99	100	401

The table shows that nearly 48 per cent of the women were married between the ages of 15-19 years, followed by 32 per cent of the women who were married between the ages of 8-14 years. Very few of the women (12%) were married either in their early or mid twenties.

It has been found that almost 62 per cent of the women in Sultanpur were married by 15-19 years of age. Only 14 per cent of the women were married in their twenties. Nearly a third of the women in Kapgari were married by the age of 8-14 years, and 41 per cent were married between the age of 15-19, whereas only about 16 per cent were married in their twenties. However, 13 per cent said they did not remember their age at marriage. Almost a quarter of the women in Motipur were married very young, between the age of 8-14, and 45 per cent were married by 15-19 years of age. Only 13 per cent of the women were married in their twenties. Quite a large proportion of the surveyed women (21%) said that they did not remember their age at marriage. A majority of the women started living with their husbands immediately after marriage in most cases.

Certain communities and tribes in India practice cross-cousin marriages or consanguineous marriages. This basically prohibits the clan/tribe members from marrying outside the lineage/clan or tribe and keeps the wealth of the family within the family circle itself. This kind of marriage rule still holds true for some of the tribal groups and the Muslims of India, and were found to exist in the study villages amongst certain groups of people.

In the tribal village of Motipur, three women were married to their own blood relatives; two of them were married to their first cousin on their father's side, and another was married to some other blood relation. The Muslims of village Kapgari too, followed this practice. Three women were related to their husbands before they were married to them. One woman was married to her first cousin on her father's side and the remaining two were married to other blood relations.

In village Santoshpur almost a quarter (25%) of the surveyed women were married to their own blood relatives. Around 12 women were married to their first cousin on their father's side, and ten of them were married to a first cousin on their mother's side, and the rest were either married to a second cousin or some other blood relation.

The Muslim and the tribal community of village Sultanpur too, followed consanguineous marriage rules. Nineteen of the surveyed women were married to their own blood relations, out of which 13 were first cousins on their father's side and five were first cousins on their mother's side.

Education

Gender bias in education is most pronounced in South Asia and the disparity between the educational levels of men and women is particularly pronounced in the rural areas, where about half of all married women are illiterate compared to their husbands. Generally, female illiteracy is more prevalent amongst the Muslim women and the tribal women. Just over a third of the total surveyed women (38%), ever attended school while 56 per cent of the males (partners of the surveyed women), had some sort of formal schooling or attended school for a certain period of time. Refer to table 4.3 more for details.

Table 4.3:   **Percentage schooling (Females and Males)**

VILLAGE	EVER ATTENDED SCHOOL (FEMALES)			EVER ATTENDED SCHOOL (MALES)		
	YES	NO	TOTAL	YES	NO	TOTAL
MOTIPUR (Tribal)	10	92	102	35	67	102
KAPGARI (Hindu)	47	53	100	72	28	100
SANTOSHPUR (Muslim)	40	59	99	48	51	99
SULTANPUR (Developed)	54	46	100	68	32	100
TOTAL	151 (37.65%)	250 (62.34%)	401	223 (55.61%)	178 (44.38%)	401

Table 4.3 shows that the women of village Sultanpur had the highest percentage of school attendance (54%), closely followed by 47 per cent of the women from village Kapgari. In the case of the men, village Kapgari (72%), had the highest percentage of formal schooling, followed by men from village Sultanpur (68%). The least amount of formal schooling in both the cases of men and women was found in the tribal village of Motipur, where only 10 per cent of the women and 35 per cent of the men ever attended school. However, in village Santoshpur, there was less difference between the schooling of men and women. The table shows that 40 per cent of the surveyed women had attended school as opposed to only 48 per cent of the males.

Village Sultanpur ranks first amongst all the other villages in school attendance by total number of persons, both males and females, followed by village Kapgari, and Santoshpur and then by Motipur. The school attendance rate in Motipur was 22 per cent and in Santoshpur it was 44 per cent. The highest school attendance rate was in Sultanpur which was almost 61 per cent, and in Kapgari it was nearly 60 per cent.

The highest grade completed by the surveyed women was the secondary level of schooling (71 as opposed to 69 who went to primary school), that is, most of the surveyed women attended school up to grade 6-10, and their partners too completed secondary level of schooling. Refer to table 4.4 for more information on highest grade completed by both the women and men of the survey population.

Table 4.4:   **Highest grade completed by males and females (Percentage)**

GRADE COMPLETED (males and females)	MOTIPUR (Tribal)		KAPGARI (Hindu)		SANTOSHPUR (Muslim)		SULTANPUR (Developed)		TOTAL	
	FEMALE	MALE	FEMALE	MALE	FEMALE	MALE	FEMALE	MALE	FEMALE	MALE
NO SCHOOLING	92	67	53	28	59	51	46	32	250 (62.34%)	178 (44.38%)
1-5 (PRIMARY)	4	14	26	25	18	14	21	36	69 (17.20%)	89 (22.19%)
6-10 (SEC.)	6	16	17	33	20	28	28	18	71 (17.70%)	95 (23.69%)
11-12 (H. SEC.)	-	3	-	5	2	1	2	7	4 (4.99%)	16 (3.99%)
GRADE 13 +	-	2	4	5	-	4	-	1	4 (4.99%)	12 (2.99%)
OTHER	-	-	-	4	-	1	3	6	3 (0.74%)	11 (2.74%)
TOTAL	102	102	100	100	99	99	100	100	401	401

The table shows that more men and women had completed secondary level of education in all villages, except Sultanpur, followed by primary level. In village Sultanpur, 36 per cent of the men had completed primary schooling and only 18 per cent had completed secondary schooling.

In the case of surveyed women, a higher number of women had completed secondary school with the exception of women from village Kapgari. Only about 26 per cent of the women in village Kapgari had completed primary level of schooling and 17 per cent secondary schooling. The figure is reversed in the other villages where a slightly higher number of women had had secondary education as opposed to the women from village Kapgari.

Literacy Levels

Though around 56 per cent of the males and 38 per cent of the surveyed women attended school, more than this could read and write. This could possibly be because of the adult literacy programme organised and run by many voluntary and government agencies in the villages. Women from villages Motipur, Kapgari and Santoshpur could read and write if they had attended school or had a formal education. However, some of the women of village

Sultanpur said that they could read and write although they had not had any formal schooling. Similarly some males from villages Kapgari and Sultanpur, could both read and write without having any formal schooling. Table 4.5 gives more details.

Table 4.5: **Ability to read and write (Females and Males)**

VILLAGE	READ AND WRITE (FEMALE)		NO SCHOOLING (F)	READ AND WRITE (MALE)		NO SCHOOLING (M)
	YES	NO		YES	NO	
MOTIPUR (Tribal)	10	92	92	35	67	67
KAPGARI (Hindu)	47	53	53	76	24	28
SANTOSHPUR (Muslim)	40	59	59	48	51	51
SULTANPUR (Developed)	77	23	46	82	18	32
TOTAL	174	227	250	241	160	178
	(43.39%)	(56.60%)	(62.34%)	(60.09%)	(39.90%)	(44.38%)

The table shows that almost a quarter of the women from village Sultanpur who had not attended school could read and write (54% of the surveyed women had attended school). This could probably be because of the ready availability and accessibility of adult schools within the village. In the case of males from villages Sultanpur and Kapgari, 14 per cent and 4 per cent of the respective men could read and write without having any schooling (in village Sultanpur 68% had attended schools and in village Kapgari 72% had some form of schooling). Therefore, the total literacy rate of the study population is 52 per cent. The male literacy rate is obviously higher (60%) than the female literacy rate (43%), because of the gender bias in education.

Utilisation of Mass Media

Though a large proportion of women did not work outside of the home for economic gain, most women still worked as hard as their male counterparts both within and outside the home. Hence, these women hardly ever had any spare time in which to relax or listen to the radio, go to the cinema and so on. When the women were asked what they did in their spare time, replies were similar. Most of them said that they sew, knit, made quilts and blankets, weave mats, etc. Very few women ever read the newspapers or listened to the radio or watched television or went to the cinema during their spare time, as only 40 per cent of the households surveyed had access to a radio or televisions (8%) (details in chapter 3).

The study shows that an overwhelming 96 per cent of the women from village Motipur never read the newspapers, as the majority of them can not read. However, nine percent listened to the radio daily and another nine per cent listened sometimes. As a majority of the households surveyed did not have a radio 84 per cent never listened to the radio. Out of 102 surveyed women from Motipur, four per cent watched television everyday, and two per cent watched it occasionally. But almost 31 per cent went to the cinema at least once or twice a month, and 69 per cent of the women said, they never had enough time to go to the cinema, though the cinema is close to the village.

In village Kapgari nearly 79 per cent of the women did not bother with the newspapers, eight per cent read one almost daily and 13 per cent said whenever they found time to relax, they read the papers. Almost 39 per cent of the surveyed women from Kapgari listened to the radio regularly, and 13 per cent listened sometimes while working or doing some household chore. Only nine per cent of the women mentioned that they watched television everyday, and five per cent watched it occasionally (most of the surveyed households do not have a television set).

In village Santoshpur only five per cent of the women read the papers daily, 21 per cent listened to the radio everyday and 15 per cent watched television regularly. However, a quarter of the surveyed women (24%) went to the cinema at least once or twice a month. In village Sultanpur, 10 per cent of the surveyed women read the newspapers daily, 41 per cent listened to the radio everyday and 34 per cent watched television daily. More than half of the surveyed women (57%) went to the cinema almost three to four times a month or whenever they had some free time. For details see table 4.6.

Table 4.6:   **Utilisation of mass media by women**

VILLAGE	READ NEWSPAPERS			LISTEN TO THE RADIO			WATCH TELEVISION			CINEMA	
	YES	NO	SOME	YES	NO	SOME	YES	NO	SOME	YES	NO
TRIBAL	4	96	2	9	84	9	4	96	2	32	70
HINDU	8	79	13	39	48	13	9	86	5	-	100
MUSLIM	5	85	9	21	58	20	15	65	19	28	71
DEVELOPED	10	90	-	41	58	1	34	64	2	57	43
	27	350	24	110	248	43	62	311	28	117	284
	(6.73%)	(87.28%)	(5.98%)	(27.43%)	(61.84%)	(10.72%)	(15.46%)	(77.55%)	(6.98%)	(29.17%)	(70.82%)

The table shows that compared to the women of other villages, the women from village Sultanpur and Kapgari read more papers and listen to the radio. A higher proportion of the women from village Sultanpur in comparison with other villages utilise the mass media. In village Santoshpur more women go to the cinema and watch television than read the papers or listen to the radio. In village Motipur, a greater proportion of the women normally only go to the cinema.

Primary Occupation of the Surveyed Population

Though all the study villages were basically rural and agricultural, the primary occupation of the people varied considerably. Table 4.7 presents more detailed information.

Table 4.7: **Main occupation of the husbands (Percentage)**

PRIMARY OCCUPATION OF SURVEYED MEN	MOTIPUR (Tribal)	KAPGARI (Hindu)	SANTOSHPUR (Muslim)	SULTANPUR (Developed)	TOTAL
LABOURER (Agricultural and Manual)	42	16	35	30	123 (30.59%)
FARMER	39	30	3	8	80 (19.90%)
BUSINESS	7	33	38	22	100 (24.87%)
SERVICE	10	21	10	30	71 (17.66%)
FISHERMAN/SHEPHERD/SNAKE CHARMER	4	-	6	-	10 (2.48%)
CARPENTER/MASON	-	-	2	5	7 (1.74%)
RICKSHAW PULLER	-	-	1	3	4 (0.99%)
LAWYER	-	-	1	2	3 (0.74%)
PRIEST	-	-	2	-	2 (0.49%)
N.A.	-	-	2	-	2 (0.49%)
TOTAL	102	100	100	100	402

A majority of the males of village Motipur were working as labourers (manual/agricultural). More than a third were farmers and cultivators, and a few were in white-collar jobs. Nearly a third of the males of village Kapgari were engaged in small scale business, and about 30 per cent were farmers and cultivators. Almost a quarter of the men were holding jobs as either teachers, clerks and bank tellers, in the postal department and so on, and a small proportion were primarily working as labourers.

Even though the village of Santoshpur is basically agricultural, the primary occupation of the surveyed population was quite varied, and was not related to agriculture. More than a third of the surveyed men had their own small business, and more than a third also worked as labourers. A very small percentage of men were engaged in white-collar jobs, and the rest either worked as carpenters, rickshaw-pullers, masons and so on. In Sultanpur, quite a large population primarily worked as labourers and a similar proportion were also employed in various other white-collar jobs. About a quarter of the surveyed population had their own small business, and only a negligible proportion of the population primarily depended on farming and cultivation. The rest were employed in a variety of other occupations.

Both the villages of Motipur and Santoshpur have only about 10 per cent of the surveyed population in the service sector. This is because a large proportion of the men in these two villages are illiterate The table further indicates that the population of Motipur and Kapgari are to a large extent dependent on agriculture. Whilst the population of Sultanpur are dependent on service and small-scale businesses because of their proximity to the city and district towns.

The occupation of the surveyed women too, varied a great deal with regards to caste, tribe, religion, income level, and so on. Table 4.8 details more information.

Table 4.8:   **Primary occupation of the surveyed women**

MAIN OCCUPATION OF SURVEYED WOMEN	MOTIPUR (Tribal)	KAPGARI (Hindu)	SANTOSHPUR (Muslim)	SULTANPUR (Developed)	TOTAL
HOUSEWIFE	59	95	84	58	296 (74.55%)
LABOURER (Agricultural and Manual)	23	1	5	25	54 (13.46%)
FARMING	12	-	-	7	19 (4.73%)
BUSINESS	2	2	4	2	10 (2.49%)
SERVICE	-	2	1	5	8 (1.99%)
MAID SERVANTS	-	-	4	3	7 (1.74%)
MAT WEAVING	6	-	-	-	6 (1.49%)
DAI/TBA	-	-	1	-	1 (0.24%)
TOTAL	102	100	99	100	401

A majority of the women from all the study villages gave housewife as their primary occupation. In addition 42 per cent of the women from villages Sultanpur and Motipur worked outside home for economic gain. This was in contrast to 95 per cent of the women in Kapgari and 84 per cent in Santoshpur who were not gainfully employed. A small number of women from all villages were engaged in running their own small scale business. Moreover, a small number of women also worked in blue-collar/white-collar jobs.

Income

The income levels of the surveyed population are of course dependent on the types and kinds of occupation, and accordingly the income levels varied a great deal. The economic status of village Sultanpur was the best amongst all the other surveyed villages, and village Motipur was the worst. See table 4.9 for more details.

Table 4.9: **Total monthly income of the surveyed population**

TOTAL MONTHLY INCOME PER PERSON IN EACH HOUSEHOLD (RUPEES)	MOTIPUR (Tribal)	KAPGARI (Hindu)	SANTOSHPUR (Muslim)	SULTANPUR (Developed)	TOTAL
25 RUPEES TO 150 (LOW INCOME RANGE)	67	50	40	2	159 (39.55%)
Rs 151 TO 350 (MIDDLE INCOME)	30	33	26	55	144 (35.82%)
Rs. 351 TO 501 & MORE (HIGH INCOME RANGE)	5	17	34	43	99 (24.62%)
TOTAL	102	100	100	100	402

The data reveals a great disparity between the income levels of the surveyed villages. Village Sultanpur is the best in terms of income levels of the population as compared to the other villages. The poorest of all is Motipur. Overall a majority of the population from all villages (40%) belonged to the low income group range (Rupees 25 to 150), followed by 36 per cent in the middle income group (Rupees 151 to 350), and about a quarter in the high income group of Rupees 351 or more.

The overall socio-economic and socio-cultural development of the study villages shows that Sultanpur is quite advanced in terms of female and male education, awareness and utilisation of the mass media, more women in the paid work force, comparatively higher age at marriage for both women and men, occupation of men, income levels, and so on as opposed to Motipur. The villages Kapgari and Santoshpur are quite similar in almost every aspect of socio-economic developments and conditions with the sole exception of education of women and men, which may be due to the different religious beliefs in these two villages.

Conclusion

Women's health status is very much dependent on the socio-economic condition of the household and accordingly the health status of the women vary considerably. The findings of the study suggests that the social conditions and cultural factors affects a woman's health status more than any other variable. It can be said that tradition and culture play a much more dominant role with regards age at marriage. A significant link exists between socio-economic development, particularly women's development, and health care behaviour and utilisation. Furthermore, socio-economic status and religion was found to play a crucial role in influencing all the variables in the study and illustrates the significance of socio-economic development and health of women.

Utilisation of Health Care Services and Family Planning

Salma is 25 years old and is a mother of three, two boys and a girl. She was married when she was 13 years old and has been married for the past 12 years. She separated from her husband seven years ago as he took another wife. I met Salma during my field work in West Bengal in late 1993.

Salma's health care utilisation and behaviour is typical of the rural women in India. For any kind of illness she normally utilises all the possible available medical and non-medical facilities within the village. For certain kind of ailments like the ones caused by evil eyes, spirits, foul wind and so on, she primarily depends on the '*Ojha*' for '*Jhar-Phoonk*'. But if the illness still persists, she visits the village quack for medicines. Even if this fails, she visits a Homeopath doctor, then depending on her health condition (worsening or not) she prefers to see a private medical practitioner. Only if the illness becomes very serious she uses the PHC or the government district hospital for treatment. She narrates how her youngest son cried persistently, and his body was swollen for a year. She thought that evil spirits had possessed her son's body, therefore she had to utilise the services of the '*Ojha*'. She says she first took her son to the PHC for treatment, but the modern medicines could not cure him. So she visited their village '*Ojha*' for treatment. The '*Ojha*' gave an amulet to be worn on the upper arm, and some holy water to drink. Even then, the illness persisted and her son kept on crying incessantly and the body swelling did not reduce. Finally, in desperation she consulted with a private allopathic medical practitioner and her son was cured within a week. Nevertheless, she still has faith in the '*Ojha*' and also strongly believes in the super-natural beings. She says she does not have any personal experience, but she heard stories from other villagers about super-natural beings and she believes that these beings can cause a lot of problems and ill-health which cannot be cured by going to a hospital, but can only be cured by the '*Ojha*'.

The literature reveals that utilisation of health services is positively influenced by factors such as female literacy and political awareness. But the literature also suggests that the mere provision of services does not always necessarily lead to their better utilisation (Jain 1985; Cassen, 1982). The present study

107

found that a large percentage of both women and men were aware of the essential and different kinds of services provided by the PHCs, and they primarily utilise the services for either family planning, or to treat common illness, or for immunisation purposes.

The focal point of this chapter is on the utilisation of available health care resources and family planning in the study villages. The general health care utilisation pattern, behaviour, perception and awareness regarding different types of ailments and illness among different groups of people were studied in order to assess the health seeking behaviour of the study population.

Utilisation of Different Means of Treatment

The above case study illustrates that women in rural India have immense faith in the supernatural, evil spirits, foul winds, evil eyes, and so on. For certain kind of illness both for children and adults alike, traditional healers or unlicensed and unqualified practitioners are preferred. The belief in the *Ojha* or other medical systems and alternative systems of cure intensifies more so, because, most of the times, even if a patient is brought to a PHC, the patient is not cured because of unavailability of medicines and essential drugs, shortage of health personnel and staff, long waiting time at the health centres, unsuitable timings of the health centres, discourteous behaviour of the PHC staff, are some of the deterrent for not using the services of the PHCs. Moreover, the poor villagers often do not have enough money to buy essential drugs from a drug store which are quite expensive.

Utilisation of Services Provided by the Primary Health Centres

The health seeking behaviour or utilisation of available health care services are quite different in the villages studied. In Motipur, the villagers tend to use the PHC in case of both major and minor illness, while in the other three areas, they prefer a private doctor to a PHC or government hospital. Though medical pluralism is flourishing in all the study villages, it is more extensive in Santoshpur and Motipur.

A majority of the women knew that the PHC provided family planning services, maternal and child health services, and other related services. But most of the women were ignorant of the fact that the PHC also provided essential drugs. The women in Motipur and Kapgari did not know anything about the distribution of essential drugs. This is because most of the times medicines and drugs are not available at the PHCs and the villagers invariably end up buying medicines from a drug store. Only nine per cent of the women in Santoshpur and 17 per cent in Sultanpur were aware that the PHC also distributed essential drugs. See table 5.1, for more details.

Table 5.1:   **Percentage aware of services provided by the PHC**

VILLAGE	F.P. SERVICES	MCH SERVICES	IMMUNISATION	TREATMENT	ESSENTIAL DRUGS
MOTIPUR (Tribal, N_1 = 102)	79	81	75	66	-
KAPGARI (Hindu, N_2 = 100)	87	84	94	80	-
SANTOSHPUR (Muslim, N_3 = 100)	95	97	94	94	9
SULTANPUR (Developed, N_4 =100)	92	74	25	89	17
TOTAL (N_T = 402)	353 (87.81%)	336 (83.58%)	288 (71.64%)	329 (81.84%)	26 (6.46%)

The findings reveal that in almost all the villages, except Sultanpur, nearly everyone used the PHC at some point in time. However, the villagers of Sultanpur preferred the district government hospital to that of their village PHC. A majority of the surveyed people used the facilities of the PHC for either family planning services, or to treat common illness, or for immunisation services. See table 5.2.

Table 5.2:   **Percent ever used the existing facilities**

VILLAGE	PHC	SUB-CENTRE	GOVERNMENT HOSPITAL	PRIVATE HOSPITAL/ CLINIC
MOTIPUR (Tribal, N_1 = 102)	100	6	44	40
KAPGARI (Hindu, N_2 = 100)	81	31	51	74
SANTOSHPUR (Muslim, N_3 = 100)	99	13	40	72
SULTANPUR (Developed, N_4 =100)	7	6	89	62
TOTAL (N_T = 402)	286 (71.14%)	56 (13.93%)	224 (55.72%)	248 (61.69%)

It is clear from the table that with increasing economic and social mobility, the preference for treatment changes drastically. It has been observed in the study villages that the economically stable and better off people also have access to various means of transportation and communication facilities, and prefer to travel either to the district town or city in case of medical emergency or need. Most economically better-off families in the study villages prefer to consult a private medical practitioner because they believe the treatment given by the PHC is not good enough to cure any major ailments.

The villagers of Kapgari, Santoshpur and Sultanpur are economically better off than those of Motipur and hence prefer to consult with a private doctor in case of major ailments. Nearly all the surveyed population feel that since the PHC and/or the government hospitals are free, the treatment and the medicines prescribed or given will not cure the illness. Therefore they like to consult with a private doctor and feel that they are getting their money's worth. Nonetheless, the villagers of the study area do utilise the services of the PHC/government hospital for minor and major ailments and in emergencies. As a majority of the surveyed villagers experienced some sort of problem in seeking treatment from the village PHC, they prefer to consult with either private practitioners or visit the nearest district government hospital for treatment. See table 5.3.

Table 5.3:   Percent faced problems in seeking treatment from PHC

VILLAGE	YES	NO	TOTAL
MOTIPUR (Tribal, N_1 = 102)	53	49	102
KAPGARI (Hindu, N_2 = 100)	60	40	100
SANTOSHPUR (Muslim, N_3 = 100)	85	15	100
SULTANPUR (Developed, N_4 =100)	12	88	100
TOTAL (N_T = 402)	210 (52.23%)	192 (47.76%)	402

The villagers in Sultanpur did not face much difficulty in seeking treatment from the PHC, because the people of this village often utilised the facilities of the district government hospital or sought treatment from a private doctor. But in all the other villages more than half of the population experienced problems and difficulties in obtaining treatment from their respective PHCs.

Almost 60 per cent of the surveyed population from village Kapgari reported that they had encountered problems and difficulties in seeking treatment from their village PHC. They said that the doctor was never on duty and never available, there were never any medicines at the centre, and the opening hours of the health centre were not suitable, as it was open only in the morning between 7:30 AM-10:30 AM.

Though 85 per cent of the surveyed population from village Santoshpur faced problems in seeking treatment from their village PHC, nonetheless, they utilised its services. Their major complaint was that most of the essential medicines were never available, and medicines were always in short supply. In Motipur 53 per cent of the population said that the major problem they encountered in seeking treatment from their village PHC was that the medicines were never available and they were too poor to buy medicines from pharmacists, and further added that doctors sometimes demanded money for better treatment and medicines.

The most universal and common complaint by a majority of the surveyed population was that of 'medicines are never available' at the PHC, followed by discourteous behaviour of the staff and health personnel, doctors never available, doctors demand money for better treatment, and so on. See table 5.4 for details.

Table 5.4: **Percent encountered problems at the PHC**

VILLAGE	MEDS. NOT AVAILABLE	DISCOURTEOUS BEHAVIOUR	DOCTORS & MEDS. NEVER AVAILABLE	LONG WAITING TIME	TOTAL
MOTIPUR (Tribal, N_1 = 102)	40	1	1	-	42
KAPGARI (Hindu, N_2 = 100)	13	23	11	-	47
SANTOSHPUR (Muslim, N_3 = 100)	79	-	-	-	79
SULTANPUR (Developed, N_4 =100)	-	2	-	4	6
TOTAL (N_T = 402)	132 (75.86%)	26 (14.94%)	12 (6.89%)	4 (2.29%)	174(43.28%)

People of the study villages were not very happy with the services/ facilities and functioning of the PHCs. They felt that the whole administration and functioning of the PHCs was in need of an overhaul. According to them more health staff and personnel should be appointed to man the health centre at all hours. Medicines and emergency treatment should be available at all times, and the PHC should be open 24 hours a day. They also felt that the behaviour of the health staff and personnel should be more pleasant and courteous towards the villagers, and the doctors and the other health staff should be more committed to their work. Nevertheless, a third of the population surveyed were of the opinion that the PHC was giving them a satisfactory service. See table 5.5.

Table 5. 5: **Opinion regarding services provided by PHC (Percentage)**

VILLAGE	EXTREMELY GOOD	SATISFACTORY	FAIR	BAD	VERY BAD	D. K.
MOTIPUR (Tribal, N_1 = 102)	-	26	41	28	3	4
KAPGARI (Hindu, N_2 = 100)	-	11	31	40	3	15
SANTOSHPUR (Muslim, N_3 = 100)	4	58	37	-	-	1
SULTANPUR (Developed, N_4 =100)	45	42	4	2	3	3
TOTAL (N_T = 402)	49 (12.18%)	137 (34.07%)	113 (28.10%)	70 (17.41%)	9 (2.23%)	23 (5.72%)

It has already been stated that medical pluralism is quite prevalent in all four villages. Both men and women tend to explore other available alternative medicines before visiting the PHC or the government hospital for treatment. In all four villages, especially in Santoshpur, for certain kinds of illness, they seek help from the *Ojha*. If the illness is not cured after a week or so then the patient is brought to the hospital. But the villagers of Motipur also seek treatment from quacks (an unqualified practitioner of medicine), who visit their village regularly. More or less almost all the surveyed population do experiment with alternative medicines before going to a trained practitioner or to the PHC/government hospital for treatment.

Both men and women try different types of medication to cure and treat an ailment. Normally, women tend to ignore their illness and do not seek any treatment unless and until the condition becomes serious or worse. The following table reveals the health seeking behaviour of adult males in the study villages.

Table 5.6(a):   Health care utilisation by adult males (Percentage)

HEALTH CARE UTILISATION	MOTIPUR (Tribal, $N_1 = 102$)	KAPGARI (Hindu, $N_2 = 100$)	SANTOSHPUR (Muslim, $N_3 = 100$)	SULTANPUR (Developed, $N_4 = 100$)	TOTAL ($N_T = 402$)
TRADITIONAL HOME REMEDIES	1	1	1	3	6 (1.49%)
WESTERN MEDICINE AT HOME	1	5	10	1	17 (4.22%)
PHC/GOVT. HOSPITAL	95	66	45	84	290 (72.13%)
PRIVATE DOCTOR	13	39	17	67	136 (33.83%)
HOMEOPATH DOCTOR	6	11	11	1	29 (7.21%)
OTHER	-	-	25	1	26 (6.46%)

The table reveals that almost three-fourths of the male population visited either the village PHC or the nearest government hospitals in case of any illness or ailment. Most of the surveyed men did not try any other alternative treatment at home before visiting the health centres for treatment. However, quite a few Muslim men from Santoshpur did try other alternative methods of treatment before finally visiting a trained medical practitioner. The data reveals that about 10 per cent of the men from Santoshpur tried western medicine at home in case of minor ailments before visiting the health centre, whereas, 11 per cent tried homeopathic medicines first. Besides, a quarter of the men believed in "other" methods of treatment, which normally meant visiting a *Ojha* or a *Moulvi* (Priest) to cure any physical ailment. Nevertheless, 45 per cent of the men visited the PHC or the government hospital, and 17 consulted with a private doctor immediately in case of any problems without exploring any other possibilities and alternatives.

Almost all the men from the socio-economically developed village of Sultanpur did not believe in any alternative medical treatment. In case of any physical discomfort or illness 84 per cent straight away visited the district government hospital or the PHC, and 67 per cent preferred to consult with a private doctor. Only about three per cent of the men tried traditional home remedies first before visiting a doctor. This could probably be because of the higher level of literacy and educational attainment of the men from this village and more knowledge and awareness about modern medicines because of improved transportation and communication facilities and also due to the proximity to the district town and the city.

Even in Kapgari, 66 per cent of the surveyed men depended either on the government hospital or the PHC, and 39 per cent on the private medical sector for treatment of their illness, without trying any other modes of treatment and cure. Nevertheless, 11 per cent tried homeopathy first before visiting an allopathic doctor, and five per cent experimented with western medicines at home before consulting a trained physician.

Similarly, the tribal men of Motipur also did not explore other means of treatment, and 95 per cent opted to visit the village PHC or the government hospital in case of any ailments. Those few relatively well-to-do households preferred to consult with a private doctor in case of illness. About six per cent of the men tried homeopathy first before visiting a western doctor. Though a large proportion of men from all the study villages opt for treatment from their health centres or the government hospitals or private clinics, quite a few men from the village of Santoshpur do try and explore other modes of treatment before going to a trained practitioner. This could possibly be because a large number of men from this village are illiterate and believe in supernatural beings and have immense faith in the 'other' methods of treatment. The tribal men from village Motipur are also illiterate, but they utilise the services of the PHC because it is free, and any other method of treatment costs money (even the ones associated with the supernatural).

Table 5.6 (b):   Health care utilisation by adult females (Percentage)

HEALTH CARE UTILISATION	MOTIPUR (Tribal, N_1=102)	KAPGARI (Hindu, N_2=100)	SANTOSHPUR (Muslim, N_3=100)	SULTANPUR (Developed, N_4=100)	TOTAL (N_T= 402)
TRADITIONAL HOME REMEDIES	3	4	2	2	11 (2.73%)
WESTERN MEDICINE AT HOME	1	5	9	2	17 (4.22%)
PHC/GOVT. HOSPITAL	90	64	43	85	282 (70.14%)
PRIVATE DOCTOR	12	36	3	58	109 (27.11%)
HOMEOPATH DOCTOR	5	6	23	7	41 (10.19%)
OTHER	2	5	30	1	38 (9.45%)

Nearly 70 per cent of the total surveyed women utilised the services of the health centres when ill. However, this was their last choice in quite a few cases, after they had tried the various other methods of available treatment. The health care utilisation behaviour of the women from village Santoshpur is very similar to their male counterparts. Almost a third of the women from this village tried the "other" methods of treatment first. Almost a quarter of the women initially tried homeopathic treatment, followed by nine per cent who administered western medicine at home, and two per cent opted for traditional home remedies for cure and treatment, before visiting and consulting a trained medical practitioner. About 43 per cent went immediately to the village PHC or the government hospital and three per cent were visited by private doctor as opposed to 17 per cent of the men of this village.

There is not much difference in the utilisation of health care services by men and women of village Sultanpur. The utilisation of health services by women is almost similar to that of men except that seven per cent of the surveyed women first try homeopathy as opposed to one per cent of the males. A majority of the women (85%) visit the district hospital in case of illness and 58 per cent consult with a private doctor immediately. About two per cent each first try western medicines at home and traditional home remedies before going to a health centre.

Whereas in village Kapgari 64 percent of the surveyed women utilised the services of the health centres, and 36 per cent consulted with private doctors at the first instant in case of any ailments. However, six per cent tried homeopathic treatment first, five percent took western medicines at home first and four per cent explored with traditional home remedies before visiting a trained doctor. About five per cent believed in the powers of supernatural and sought treatment from traditional healers, depending on the nature and type of ailment.

However, almost 90 per cent of the tribal women of village Motipur said that in case of any physical problems, they immediately visited the village PHC for treatment. Five per cent of the women tried homeopathy first, and three per cent traditional home remedies before visiting a trained physician. About 12 per cent relatively well-to-do households preferred to consult with a private doctor in case of illness. Two per cent also visited the *Ojha* first for treatment before going to the PHC.

A large proportion of the surveyed women from all the study villages opted for treatment from their health centres or the government hospitals or private clinics. Nevertheless, some women from village Santoshpur explored other modes of treatment before going to a trained practitioner. This could possibly be because of illiteracy and lack of knowledge amongst the women and belief in supernatural beings. Even though the tribal women from village Motipur are also illiterate, they utilised the services of the PHC because it is free, and all other kinds of treatment cost money.

Men are given more importance than women in case of an illness in the family. A mere one per cent of the men in the study population try any sort of traditional home remedies as opposed to three per cent of women. Ten per cent of the surveyed women go for homeopathic treatment as opposed to seven per cent of the men. A higher percentage of women try out the different available options more readily than men. The reason behind this is that the men are the bread winners of the family and cannot afford to be ill for a long period, hence medical attention is sought for males more readily than women.

The perception of different ailments in the study population is almost similar to one another. The perception of major and minor ailments is generally based on their personal experiences or that of their friends or relatives or neighbours. In all the four villages, the people listed dysentery and diarrhoea to be a major ailment. But a majority of the people in the study population are unaware of ailments such as diabetes, blood pressure and so on. There were differing views on other illness and ailments. See table 5.7 (a) for more details.

Table 5.7 (a):   **Perception of major illness (Percentage)**

PERCEPTION	MOTIPUR (Tribal, N_1=102)	KAPGARI (Hindu, N_2=100)	SANTOSHPUR (Muslim, N_3=100)	SULTANPUR (Developed, N_4=100)	TOTAL (N_T= 402)
BLOOD PRESSURE	-	5	19	6	30 (7.46%)
DIABETES	1	6	14	-	21 (5.22%)
INFECTIONS	2	4	29	1	36 (8.95%)
TUBERCULOSIS	30	53	50	6	139 (34.57%)
CHOLERA	29	62	54	2	147 (36.56%)
DYSENTERY & DIARRHOEA	86	88	89	68	331 (82.33%)
BRONCHITIS	9	19	39	3	70 (17.41%)
MALARIA	41	49	9	1	100 (24.87%)
TETANUS	7	19	13	1	40 (9.95%)
PNEUMONIA	10	15	2	1	28 (6.96%)

Numerous studies have shown that diarrhoea is associated with infant and child deaths, particularly among infants not breast-fed or during supplementation and weaning (Gray, 1989). Diarrhoea is a major cause of morbidity and mortality in young children. It has been estimated that about 10 per cent of the deaths in the first year of life and about 14 per cent in ages (1-4) are due to gastro-enteritis (Government of India, 1988). About 50 per cent of infants and 20 per cent of pre-school children suffer from acute diarrhoeal problems. Every year, about 1.5 million children under five die because of diarrhoea, of whom 60 per cent die of dehydration (Sinha, 1990).

As perception of an ailment is based on personal experience, the surveyed population classified and categorised major and minor ailments accordingly. It was agreed by all the study population that headaches, coughs and colds, fevers and so on were minor ailments and did not need any treatment. According to them, these ailments took their own course and time and eventually cured themselves without any medical intervention. See table 5.7 (b).

Table 5.7 (b):   Perception of minor illness (Percentage)

PERCEPTION (MINOR ILLNESS)	MOTIPUR (Tribal, N_1=102)	KAPGARI (Hindu, N_2=100)	SANTOSHPUR (Muslim, N_3=100)	SULTANPUR (Developed, N_4=100)	TOTAL (N_T= 402)
HEAD ACHES	70	64	66	13	213 (52.98%)
STOMACH ACHES	-	38	5	6	49 (12.18%)
BACK ACHES	33	34	16	7	90 (22.38%)
CUTS & WOUNDS	57	49	24	2	132 (32.83%)
INFLUENZA	13	26	18	17	74 (18.40%)
COUGH & COLD	70	83	78	85	316 (78.60%)
FEVER	81	68	60	76	285 (70.89%)
RASHES	21	17	4	17	59 (14.67%)
BODY ACHE	12	14	5	4	35 (8.70%)
SCABIES	14	4	1	1	20 (4.97%)
OTHER	2	-	8	11	21 (5.22%)

Almost half of the study population sought treatment for dysentery and diarrhoea, followed by bronchitis, malaria, cholera and tuberculosis, which they consider to be major illnesses. It seems dysentery and diarrhoea are the most dreaded and severe ailment the study population frequently encounters.

Table 5.8 (a):   Percentage seeking treatment for major ailments

TREATMENT (MAJOR AILMENTS)	MOTIPUR (Tribal, N_1=204)	KAPGARI (Hindu, N_2=200)	SANTOSHPUR (Muslim, N_3=200)	SULTANPUR (Developed, N_4=200)	TOTAL (N_T= 804)
BLOOD PRESSURE	-	2 (1%)	7 (3.5%)	2 (1%)	11 (1.36%)
DIABETES	-	-	5 (2.5%)	-	5 (0.62%)
INFECTIONS	4 (1.96%)	1 (0.5%)	33 (16.5%)	-	38 (4.72%)
TUBERCULOSIS	2 (0.98%)	1 (0.5%)	20 (10%)	2 (1%)	25 (3.10%)
CHOLERA	3 (1.47%)	3 (1.5%)	24 (12%)	-	30 (3.73%)
DYSENTERY & DIARRHOEA	42 (20.58%)	4 (20.5%)	71 (35.5%)	39 (19.5%)	193 (24.0%)
BRONCHITIS	9 (4.41%)	12 (6%)	37 (18.5%)	9 (4.5%)	67 (8.33%)
MALARIA	13 (6.37%)	16 (8%)	4 (2%)	4 (2%)	37 (4.60%)
TETANUS	7 (3.43%)	9 (4.5)	9 (4.5%)	1 (0.5%)	26 (3.23%)
PNEUMONIA	9 (4.41%)	15 (7.5%)	-	1 (0.5%)	25 (3.10%)
OTHER	-	7	(3.5%)	2 (1%)	2 (1%) 11
(1.36%)					

Table 5.8 (b) shows that though the people perceived coughs and colds, fevers, and influenza to be minor ailments, nearly one fourth of the surveyed

population sought treatment for fever. About one third sought treatment for influenza, followed by coughs and colds.

Table 5.8 (b):   **Percentage seeking treatment for minor ailments**

TREATMENT (MINOR AILMENTS)	MOTIPUR (Tribal, N_1=204)	KAPGARI (Hindu, N_2=200)	SANTOSHPUR (Muslim, N_3=200)	SULTANPUR (Developed, N_4=200)	TOTAL (N_T= 804)
HEAD ACHES	11 (5.39%)	9 (4.5%)	12 (6%)	16 (8%)	48 (5.97%)
STOMACH ACHES	8 (3.92%)	3 (1.5%)	1 (0.5%)	8 (4%)	20 (2.48%)
BACK ACHES	1 (0.49%)	1 (0.5%)	10 (5%)	4 (2%)	16 (1.99%)
CUTS & WOUNDS	3 (1.47%)	8 (4%)	33 (16.5%)	2 (1%)	46 (5.72%)
INFLUENZA	21 (10.29%)	17 (8.5%)	7 (3.5%)	9 (4.5%)	54 (6.71%)
COUGHS & COLDS	19 (9.31%)	22 (11%)	53 (26.5%)	65 (32.5%)	159 (19.77%)
FEVER	66 (32.35%)	61 (30.5%)	40 (20%)	57 (28.5%)	224 (27.86%)
RASHES	6 (2.94%)	16 (8%)	5 (2.5%)	10 (5%)	37 (4.60%)
BODY ACHE	-	2 (1%)	2 (1%)	2 (1%)	6 (0.74%)
SCABIES	4 (1.96%)	2 (1%)	3 (1.5%)	2 (1%)	11 (1.36%)
OTHER	-	-	17 (8.5%)	11 (5.5%)	28 (3.48%)

Even though a large number of people thought that treatment was not required for minor ailments, a majority of them still sought treatment for them. This may be because the medical facilities and services are readily available and free, and this encourages people to use them, even if medicines are seldom available at the health centres. This shows that people in the rural areas are very dependent on the PHCs and use them very frequently for treating minor ailments, for family planning purposes, for immunisations, and also utilise the facilities during an emergency.

General health care utilisation and behaviour of the study population was found to be varied. Medical pluralism existed in the study villages. The villagers of Motipur used the services of the PHC in case of both major and minor ailments, whereas, in the other three study villages, the surveyed population preferred to either consult with a private medical practitioner or visit the government hospital in case of any illness.

Improving Primary Health Care

Even though people use the services of the PHC as a last resort, nonetheless they use it. Therefore to enhance its image, there is a need to improve the facilities and service delivery system of the PHCs to serve the community in an effective manner. The PHCs should be open through out the day and night and medicines and essential drugs should be available at all the times. The health staff and personnel should be motivated enough to treat each patient with care and respect irrespective of their socio-economic background.

The Role of the PHCs and their Failure to Perform

The Primary Health Centre (PHC) is the core institution of the rural health services infrastructure and its basic role is essentially to provide education concerning prevailing health problems and identifying, preventing and controlling them; promotion of food supply and proper nutrition; maternal and child health care, including family planning; immunisation against the major infectious diseases; prevention and control of locally endemic diseases; treatment of common diseases and injuries; and provision of essential drugs.

However, in all the study villages it was observed that the PHCs failed to perform its duties satisfactorily. For instance, common medicines were never available at the health centres to treat minor ailments, in addition, the PHCs were unable to contain the locally endemic diseases because of lack of medicines and staff; discourteous behaviour of the health staff and personnel; long waiting time at the health centres; unsuitable timings; and in some cases the doctors were often missing from the PHCs.

In village Motipur, though the PHC doctor was present at all times, he treated the patients unkindly when they visited the health centre for treatment. However, the same doctor in his private practice treated patients with more care and respect. The whole purpose of public delivery system is defeated when the doctors do not treat patients properly and courteously at the health centres but take immense care to treat patients with care, love and patience in their illegal private practice (According to Government of India, the doctors working with the public sector are not allowed to practice their trade privately. In lieu of private practice they are given a non-practice allowance, which often is very meagre. Therefore to supplement their income they practice privately). The wages and other incentives of the public sector health delivery services personnel have to be greatly improved for total commitment and responsibility towards their office.

In village Kapgari, the PHC is just a skeletal institution as the doctor is hardly ever present, the timings (opening hours of the PHC) of the health centre is not suitable for the villagers and medicines are seldom available. Only a nurse and a health worker are available at all times at the PHC, and they are not at all amiable to the villagers and often discourteous. Therefore the villagers often choose to seek treatment from the private sector instead of the public sector.

Though the PHC in Santoshpur is well-staffed and has a bed capacity of 30 patients at any given time and is open 24 hours a day, medicines are always inadequate and in short supply. In addition, the health staff are very discourteous to the patients and do not have any patience or tolerance towards the illiterate villagers. Therefore many villagers who are economically better off prefer to consult with a private doctor since they are assured of better quality of service, care and respect in treatment.

In village Sultanpur, people consciously do not utilise the services of the PHC and prefer the district hospital for better facilities and specialist care or see a private practitioner. They refrain from visiting the PHC because of big queues and inadequate facilities.

The PHCs should train more health workers and para-medical staff from the local community who should be equipped and trained to handle and treat almost all minor diseases and locally endemic diseases. They should be deployed to provide para-medical services at the village level in an efficient and organised manner. More female health workers should be deployed to handle women's health problems at the village level and these grassroots workers should be empowered to act as referral service to the PHC level and beyond to deal with complications.

Observation of a Primary Health Centre

During my field work in a village of West Bengal in late 1993, I visited the Block primary health centre and witnessed the behaviour of the health personnel towards the villagers first hand. When a patient was brought in with severe dysentery and diarrhoea, the first thing the attending physician did was scream at the patient and his relatives for not paying attention to personal hygiene and for the delay in bringing the patient to the health centre. However, the PHC did not have any saline drip or essential drugs to give to the patient and asked the patient's relatives to buy the saline solution from the local drug store, but the relatives did not have enough money to buy the drip. The patient was left lying on the PHC floor throughout the day without any adequate treatment or attention from the health staff. It is no wonder then, that patients prefer to use either private medical sector for treatment or try alternative methods of treatment.

Family Planning and Health of Women: A Second Look

Attitude of rural women towards family planning, their knowledge, awareness and utilisation of different family planning methods are discussed here. The government's family planning programme promotes sterilisation zealously as a family planning method and the emphasis of the Indian government is more on sterilisation of women (permanent method) rather than any other reversible method. The health staff at the primary health care level are more involved with achieving family planning targets, as failure to do so is punishable. Therefore rather than promoting other methods of family planning the staff are intent on sterilisation.

Contraception

The data shows that the level of awareness regarding different types of modern family planning methods is quite high. The women in Kapgari are the most aware and knowledgeable about different kinds of family planning methods, closely followed by Santoshpur. Surprisingly, the most developed village, Sultanpur, is the one lagging behind other villages in terms of awareness and knowledge regarding different modern contraceptive methods.

The women in Sultanpur had heard about other methods, but their knowledge about condoms as an effective modern family planning method is very low as compared to the other study villages. This is because the reversible methods of family planning are not actively advertised or available at the local PHC, and moreover, the family planning methods which are zealously promoted are basically for women users. They also seemed to be less aware about male sterilisation. Only about a third of the women had ever heard about male sterilisation in the village of Sultanpur. Tables 5.9 and 5.10 presents more details.

Table 5.9:   **Percentage of women aware of different family planning methods**

VILLAGE	PILLS (%)	LOOP OR COPPER T (%)	FEMALE STERILISATION (%)
MOTIPUR (Tribal, N_1 =102)	86	83	94
KAPGARI (Hindu, N_2 =100)	99	93	99
SANTOSHPUR (Muslim, N_3 =99)	87	73	87
SULTANPUR (Developed, N_4 =100)	84	77	83
TOTAL (N_T =401)	356 (88.77%)	326 (81.29%)	363 (90.52%)

Table 5.10:   Percentage of women aware of male family planning methods

VILLAGE	CONDOMS (%)	MALE STERILISATION (%)
MOTIPUR (Tribal, N$_1$=102)	45	52
KAPGARI (Hindu, N$_2$=100)	72	93
SANTOSHPUR (Muslim, N$_3$=99)	88	57
SULTANPUR (Developed, N$_4$=100)	40	27
TOTAL (N$_T$ =401)	245 (61.09%)	229 (57.10%)

Knowledge about natural family planning methods amongst the surveyed women was almost negligible in all the four study villages. A large majority of the women had never heard of withdrawal, rhythm method, and so on. Though the level of awareness regarding different family planning methods is low in the village of Sultanpur, the percentage of women having ever used any kind of family planning methods is quite high. Refer to table 5.11.

Table 5.11:   Percentage of women ever used and currently using family planning

VILLAGE	EVER USED F.P. (%)	CURRENT USER OF F.P. (%)
MOTIPUR (Tribal, N$_1$ =102)	44	32
KAPGARI (Hindu, N$_2$ =100)	61	43
SANTOSHPUR (Muslim, N$_3$ =99)	54	48
SULTANPUR (Developed, N$_4$ =100)	62	48
TOTAL (N$_T$ =401)	221 (55.11%)	171 (42.64%)

Not much variation was found in the current users of family planning in the villages. Around 43 per cent of the surveyed women are still practising some kind of family planning method. In almost all the villages a majority of the women currently using any kind of contraceptives have been sterilised. Very few women prefer the temporary method of family planning. An overwhelming percentage of women prefer to complete the family's desired family size before using any family planning methods. Nearly all the women surveyed started a family immediately after getting married, irrespective of their age. But, a majority of them had knowledge and are aware about family planning and most of them knew from where family planning services and methods could be obtained (Refer to table 5.12).

Table 5.12:   Knowledge about where to obtain family planning services

VILLAGE	KNOW WHERE TO OBTAIN FAMILY PLANNING METHODS (%)
MOTIPUR (Tribal, N$_1$ =102)	80
KAPGARI (Hindu, N$_2$ =100)	95
SANTOSHPUR (Muslim, N$_3$ =99)	84
SULTANPUR (Developed, N$_4$ =100)	94
TOTAL (N$_T$ =401)	353 (88.02%)

Majority of the women had consulted either a doctor or a nurse before accepting and using a family planning method. This is probably because the health centres are close to the surveyed villages and the health workers and the ICDS workers working in these villages constantly encourage the women to use family planning services to limit their family size, and also advise them to consult with professionals before using any contraception. See table 5.13.

Table 5.13:   **Percentage consulting professionals before using family planning methods**

VILLAGE	% CONSULTED PROFESSIONALS BEFORE USING F.P. METHODS	%EVER USED F. P.
MOTIPUR (Tribal, N_1 =102)	35	44
KAPGARI (Hindu, N_2 =100)	50	61
SANTOSHPUR (Muslim, N_3 =99)	50	54
SULTANPUR (Developed, N_4 =100)	59	62
TOTAL (N_T =401)	194 (48.37%)	221 (55.11%)

Nearly a quarter of the women who used a family planning method experienced problems and difficulty with the use of the method (table 5.14).

Table 5.14:   **Percentage encountered problems with use of family planning methods**

VILLAGE	PROBLEMS WITH USE OF F. P. (%)	% EVER USED F. P.
MOTIPUR (Tribal, N_1 =102)	n=13 (29.54%)	44
KAPGARI (Hindu, N_2 =100)	n=9 (14.75%)	61
SANTOSHPUR (Muslim, N_3 =99)	n=13 (24.07%)	54
SULTANPUR (Developed, N_4 =100)	n=17 (27.41%)	62
TOTAL (N_T =401)	52 (23.52%)	221 (55.11%)

The most common complaint associated with the use of family planning methods in all the study villages was that of dizziness, cramps, body ache, weight gain and so on. But the universal complaint was that of dizziness. Refer to table 5.15 for the types of problems associated with the use of family planning.

Table 5.15: **Problems with use of family planning methods (Percentage)**

PROBLEMS WITH USE OF F. P.	MOTIPUR (Tribal, N_1 =44)	KAPGARI (Hindu, N_2 = 61)	SANTOSHPUR (Muslim, N_3 = 54)	SULTANPUR (Developed, N_4 = 62)	TOTAL (N_T = 221)
CRAMPS	1 (2.27%)	-	1 (1.85%)	7 (11.29%)	9 (4.07%)
DIZZINESS	8 (18.18%)	3 (4.91%)	6 (11.11%)	6 (9.67%)	23 (10.40%)
BODY ACHE	3 (6.81%)	-	2 (3.70%)	2 (3.22%)	7 (3.16%)
BLEEDING	-	-	-	1 (1.61%)	1 (0.45%)
NAUSEA AND VOMITING	7 (15.90%)	-	-	-	7 (3.16%)
WEIGHT GAIN	1 (2.27%)	-	1 (1.85%)	-	2 (0.90%)
WHITE DISCHARGE	- 1(1.63%)	-	2 (3.22%)	3 (1.35%)	3 (1.35%)
HEADACHES	10 (22.72%)	1 (1.63%)	-	1 (1.61%)	12 (5.42%)
ALLERGY	1 (2.27%)	-	-	1 (1.61%)	2 (0.90%)
BREAST TENDERNESS	1 (2.27%)	-	-	-	1 (0.45%)
OTHER	1 (2.27%)	4 (6.55%)	3 (5.55%)	2 (3.22%)	10 (4.52%)
TOTAL	33 (75%)	9 (14.75)	13 (24.07%)	22 (35.48%)	77 (34.84%)

The duration of family planning use varied between the villages. In the tribal village of Motipur, almost half of the women had been using family planning methods for less than a year. Likewise, in Santoshpur 67 per cent of the women were using some kind of family planning methods for less than a year or so. In village Sultanpur, 39 per cent of the women had been using family planning methods for more than six years. In Kapgari, nearly a third of the women had been using family planning for about two to three years. Table 5.16 presents more details.

Table 5.16: **Duration of family planning use (Percentage)**

DURATION OF F. P. USE	MOTIPUR (Tribal, N_1 =44)	KAPGARI (Hindu, N_2 = 61)	SANTOSHPUR (Muslim, N_3 = 54)	SULTANPUR (Developed, N_4 = 62)	TOTAL (N_T = 221)
LESS THAN A YEAR	22 (50%)	23 (37.70%)	36 (66.66%)	17 (27.41%)	98 44.34%)
LESS THAN TWO YEARS	9 (20.45%)	18 (29.50%)	1 (1.85%)	6 (9.67%)	34 (15.38%)
LESS THAN THREE YEARS	8 (18.18%)	14 (22.95%)	3 (5.55%)	4 (6.45%)	29 (13.12%)
LESS THAN FOUR YEARS	5 (11.36%)	6 (9.83%)	5 (9.25%)	6 (9.67%)	22 (9.95%)
LESS THAN FIVE YEARS	-	-	2 (3.70%)	5 (8.06%)	7 (3.16%)
SIX YEARS AND MORE	-	-	7 (12.96%)	24 (38.70%)	31 (14.02%)
TOTAL	44 (19.90%)	61 (27.60%)	54 (24.43%)	62 (28.05%)	221

In almost every village, a majority of the women had obtained family planning methods and services from the public sector usually from their village PHCs and/or the district government hospitals. But about three fourths of the women of village Sultanpur had obtained the methods from the district government hospital as opposed to the five per cent who had obtained it from the village PHC. See table 5.17 for further information.

Though a majority of the surveyed population had made use of the public sector in obtaining family planning services, quite a few women had opted for the private medical sector. These women undeniably come from a higher socio-economic strata of society and are inevitably more educated than their compatriots. Besides, some women also utilised other private sources in obtaining contraception.

Table 5.17:   Source of obtaining family planning methods (Percentage)

OBTAINED F. P. METHOD FROM:	MOTIPUR (Tribal, N_1 =44)	KAPGARI (Hindu, N_2 = 61)	SANTOSHPUR (Muslim, N_3 = 54)	SULTANPUR (Developed, N_4 = 62)	TOTAL (N_T = 221)
PUBLIC SECTOR					
GOVT. HOSPITAL	4 (9.09%)	11 (18.03)	4 (7.40%)	45 (72.58%)	64 (28.95%)
PHC	36 (81.81%)	30 (49.18%)	34 (62.96%)	3 (4.83%)	103 (46.60%)
SUB-CENTRE	-	-	1 (1.85%)	2 (3.22%)	3 (1.35%)
MOBILE CLINIC	-	2 (3.27%)	-	1 (1.61%)	3 (1.35%)
PRIVATE MEDICAL SECTOR					
PRIVATE HOSP./CLINIC	-	2 (3.27%)	2 (3.70%)	3 (4.83%)	7 (3.16%)
PRIVATE DOCTOR	-	-	-	3 (4.83%)	3 (1.35%)
PHARMACY/DRUGSTORE	-	6 (9.83%)	4 (7.40%)	2 (3.22%)	12 (5.42%)
OTHER PRIVATE SECTOR					
SHOP	1 (2.27%)	5 (8.19%)	7 (12.96%)	2(3.22%)	15 (6.78%)
TRADITIONAL PRACTITIONER	1 (2.27%)	1 (1.63%)	1 (1.85%)	-	3 (1.35%)
AYURVEDIC DOCTOR	1 (2.27%)	2 (3.27%)	-	-	3 (1.35%)
HOMEOPATH DOCTOR	-	-	-	1 (1.61%)	1 (0.45%)
OTHER SOURCES	1 (2.27%)	2 (3.27%)	1 (1.85%)	-	4 (1.80%)
TOTAL	44 (19.90%)	61 (27.60%)	54 (24.43%)	62 (28.05%)	221

In order to understand this data it is important to emphasise that the women of village Motipur, Kapgari and Santoshpur have faith in the traditional practitioners and healers. Even for family planning methods, some of them consult with the faith healers and traditional practitioners, who prescribe an armlet or an amulet to be worn on the upper arm to prevent conception. Needless to say, this method fails to prevent conception. Nonetheless, the surveyed women have maintained their faith in the traditional practitioners.

The women who had discontinued using family planning methods gave numerous reasons for doing so. But one of the main reasons, which was applicable to all the villages with the exception of Sultanpur, was that women wanted to have an additional child. The other reasons were related to health and other related problems. See table 5.18 for the reasons.

Table 5.18:   **Reasons for discontinuing family planning (Percentage)**

REASONS FOR DISCONTINUING F. P.	MOTIPUR (Tribal, $N_1 = 12$)	KAPGARI (Hindu, $N_2 = 18$)	SANTOSHPUR (Muslim, $N_3 = 6$)	SULTANPUR (Developed, $N_4 = 14$)	TOTAL ($N_T = 50$)
METHOD FAILED/GOT PREGNANT	-	1 (5.55%)	1 (16.66%)	3 (21.42%)	5 (10%)
LACK OF SEXUAL SATISFACTION	-	-	1 (16.66%0	2 (14.28%)	3 (6%)
CREATED MENSTRUAL PROBLEMS	3 (25%)	-	-	1 (7.14%)	4 (8%)
CREATED HEALTH PROBLEMS	3 (25%)	2 (11.11%)	1 (16.66%)	6 (42.85%)	12 (24%)
DIFFICULT TO OBTAIN METHOD	-	4 (22.22%)	-	-	4 (8%)
WANTED A CHILD	6 (50%)	9 (50%)	3 (50%)	-	18 (36%)
OTHER	-	2 (11.11%)	-	2 (14.28%)	4 (8%)
TOTAL	12 (24%)	18 (36%)	6 (12%)	14 (28%)	50

The data suggests that village Sultanpur is more advanced in terms of acceptance of family planning programmes. This can be attributed to the fact that almost three fourths of the surveyed women are literate and more than half of the surveyed women had some kind of schooling and are economically in a better position than the other study villages. In comparison only two-fifths of the women in village Santoshpur, about forty-seven percent in village Kapgari and a mere ten per cent in village Motipur are literate, and have some kind of formal schooling. Though the women of village Sultanpur did not seem to be as aware of various methods of contraception as in the other villages, but sixty-two per cent of the women had used some kind of family planning methods at some point in their lives. The duration of use of various family planning methods in Sultanpur was one of the highest as opposed to the other study villages.

It is a known fact that exposure to mass media like the radio, newspapers, television and cinema, increases knowledge and awareness about family planning messages and methods. Besides exposure to mass media, schooling also augments the overall knowledge about various important facets of life. Tests of significance was performed to find out the extent of knowledge, awareness about various family planning methods due to schooling and exposure to mass media.

The chi-square (x^2) test reveals that the relationship between utilisation of mass media and knowledge of various family planning methods is significant. The tests indicates that more women are aware about different family planning methods because of exposure to the mass media and particularly, to the print media and the radio.

Schooling of both males and females also has a significant impact on the knowledge regarding different family planning methods. The x^2 test reveals a correlation between schooling of both women and men and knowledge of various family planning methods; [$x^2 = 25.29$, P≤0.05] in case of women and [$x^2 = 17.06$, P≤0.05] in case of men. This is because schooling of even a few years and level of educational attainment increases overall awareness and knowledge. The relationship between literacy and knowledge of different family planning methods also were found to be significant [x^2=26.46, P≤0.05] in case of literate women, and in case of literate men [x^2=17.60, P≤0.05]. Therefore it can be inferred that awareness and knowledge about different family planning methods are linked and associated significantly with literacy and schooling of males and females.

However, no significant statistical relationship has been found between income, occupation and knowledge of family planning methods. Hence, the statistical significance test results reveal that awareness and knowledge of different family planning methods are to a large extent due to the exposure to mass media and communication. Furthermore, it is also due to schooling and literacy of women and men. Consequently, a significant association and relationship between schooling, literacy, exposure to mass media and knowledge of various family planning methods has been found.

Conclusion

The key findings of the study shows certain similarities and differences in health care behaviour between the villages and it was also observed that the influence of tradition and culture played a major role on certain aspects of health care behaviour. Medical pluralism was found to be flourishing in all the study villages and people switched from one medical system to another depending on affordability and time. Moreover, health care utilisation was influenced either by the perceived severity of illness, time constraint, accessibility and economic constraint.

The level of awareness regarding different types of modern family planning methods is also quite high in the study villages. Very few women prefer temporary methods of family planning. Most women prefer sterilisation and this has been the official family planning focus and target of the government. An overwhelming percentage of women preferred to complete the family's desired family size before accepting any family planning methods. The women who discontinued using temporary family planning methods did so because they wanted to have an additional child, preferably a son. The present study found that increasing levels of women's education and literacy have a positive influence on their attitude, practice and behaviour towards accepting new ideas, concepts, and utilisation of modern family planning methods.

Pregnancy and Childbirth

When Sitara was pregnant with her last child she was not allowed to go out of the house after dark because of the fear of evil spirits harming her unborn baby and also of possessing her. Her belief in the spirits and supernatural powers is very deep and strong as she herself experienced the pain of possession by the spirits. Sitara was possessed by a spirit after the delivery of her last child. During the period of her possession she was always scared and terrified of her husband and could not spend a night alone in the house on her own. She was so frightened and troubled that she would scream most of the time after dark and could not look her husband in the eye or meet his gaze. She was taken to the district town to a '*Peer Baba*' (Shaman) for treatment and exorcism. The '*Peer Baba*' said it was the foul and evil winds which had affected her and taken possession of her body. She was eventually cured of the possession by the '*Peer Baba*'. Because of her own personal experience, she believes very strongly in the supernatural and believes a woman who is pregnant or has recently given birth is very susceptible to possession by evil spirits.

Sitara delivered her youngest son at home. However, she visited the primary health centre for antenatal check-ups. But took her tetanus injections and iron/folic and acid tablets from the visiting Lady Nurse/Health Worker and not from the PHC, as all the attending physicians were males. During the entire term of her pregnancy she went only twice for her antenatal check-ups at the PHC. She did not choose to deliver at the PHC or at the government hospital because "*it is not a comfortable place and I feel inhibited, and moreover, there was no problem with my pregnancy.*" She visited the health centre for antenatal check-ups because the health workers persuaded her to do so by telling her that there might be some risk for the baby or to her health if she did not attend the antenatal clinics. Therefore she attended the prenatal clinic to have a healthy baby. Moreover, the doctors at the health centre prescribed tonics and vitamins for her which she said was good for the baby's development and growth.

This chapter deals with the knowledge, attitude, practice and behaviour of the women who were pregnant during the time of the survey and also of those women who had given birth within the last five years prior to the survey. It

127

particularly deals with the prenatal care adopted by the pregnant women, as antenatal care varies from urban to rural, between different religious groups and sects. But, utilisation of antenatal care depends to a large extent on the socio-economic and socio-cultural background of the respondents.

Prenatal Care

The survey data indicates that 41 per cent of the pregnant women of village Kapgari were visited at home during pregnancy by either a health worker, Auxiliary Nurse Midwife (ANM), or a Lady Health Visitor (LHV), from the Maternal and Child Health Care (MCH) Unit. Only a quarter of the pregnant women of village Motipur had home visits by any health personnel. Most number of home visits by health staff (51%) was observed in village Sultanpur. In village Santoshpur, a third of the pregnant women were visited at home for prenatal care. See table 6.1.

Table 6.1:   **Home visit for pregnant women by health staff**

VILLAGE	HOME VISIT FOR PREGNANT WOMEN (%)
MOTIPUR (Tribal, N_1 = 102)	25
KAPGARI (Hindu, N_2 = 100)	41
SANTOSHPUR (Muslim, N_3 = 100)	33
SULTANPUR (Developed, N_4 = 100)	51
TOTAL (N_T = 402)	150 (37.31%)

In all the surveyed villages, with the exception of village Sultanpur, the home visits were mainly accomplished during the second trimester of pregnancy. The number of home visits by health staff were almost similar in all the villages. The home visits were limited to about two to three visits during the entire term of pregnancy.

Despite home visits, a majority of the pregnant women had registered either with the village primary health centre or the district government hospital for antenatal care and check-ups. See table 6.2 for details.

Table 6.2:   **Women registered for antenatal care**

VILLAGE	PREGNANT WOMEN REGISTERED FOR ANTENATAL CARE (%)
MOTIPUR (Tribal, N_1 = 102)	70
KAPGARI (Hindu, N_2 = 100)	87
SANTOSHPUR (Muslim, N_3 = 100)	56
SULTANPUR (Developed, N_4 = 100)	85
TOTAL (N_T = 402)	298 (74.12%)

The women in Santoshpur lagged behind in registering for antenatal care. The women who had not registered for antenatal care thought antenatal care was not essential and necessary. Others were of the opinion that since they were visited at home and were given iron/folic acid tablets and tetanus injections, it was pointless to register at the health centre for a check-up. In addition, a few women were unaware of the available MCH facilities at their village health centres and hence did not register.

Most of the women who had registered for antenatal care had visited the health centre for antenatal check-ups only three times during the entire term of their pregnancy, closely followed by six times. Most of the women went for an antenatal check-up for the first time during the fifth month of pregnancy, closely followed by seventh month and the third month respectively. Very few women went for an antenatal check-up during the first trimester of pregnancy. Almost 85 per cent of the currently pregnant women (during the survey) reckoned they would register for antenatal care at a later date, and the remaining were not so sure whether they wanted to register for prenatal care and were not sure if it would benefit them. Majority of the women who had registered for antenatal care were given the iron/folic acid tablets during their pregnancy. In villages Kapgari and Motipur, they were given these tablets three times during their entire term of pregnancy, whilst in the other two villages, Santoshpur and Sultanpur, the tablets were given twice.

Nearly 70 per cent of the women had iron/folic acid tablets daily and those who had not taken the tablets said, it was because of the bad/foul smell which made them nauseous. Besides, a few women from Santoshpur reckoned that the tablets were hazardous for the baby and never took them. Three fourths of the pregnant women had taken two to three tetanus toxoid injections during their pregnancy.

Almost all the women who had registered at antenatal clinics were given very similar advice and instructions by the health personnel. Most of them were advised to keep away from heavy, strenuous, laborious and tedious chores and were advised against lifting heavy objects and things (for example, carrying water). They were also instructed to eat proper nutritious and balanced meals, and were advised to include protein, calcium, minerals and vitamins in their diet. In most of the cases the women did not follow the instructions and advice given by the health staff. Almost 81 per cent of the women in Motipur ignored the instructions and thought it to be of little value, while others stated poverty to be a major hindrance in improving their diet and food intake pattern. A third of the women in Santoshpur could not rest as advised because of lack of domestic help and poverty was cited as an obstacle in improving eating habits.

Few women also thought it was not necessary to follow the advice given by the health personnel because, they themselves had healthy babies earlier and many women in the village who had not registered for any care nor followed any advice of the health personnel had healthy babies.

Only 18 per cent of the pregnant women in Sultanpur did not follow the instructions. The reasons for not doing so were very similar to the ones given in the other villages. The most important reason was that there was no help available at home or outside to do various chores and five per cent thought it was not always necessary to follow the advice given by the doctors. In Kapgari nearly two-thirds (64%) of the women did not follow the instructions given by health personnel and the reason given was that there was no help available in and around the house (36%), whilst 48 per cent said they were too poor to either hire help or improve their food intake.

Illness/Sickness During Pregnancy

"I felt very dizzy during all my pregnancies, but I never thought of seeking any treatment as all the other women in the village told me it was a natural process of child bearing. Therefore, I continued with my usual tasks ignoring my physical discomfort."

Many women experience illness during pregnancy or some sort of problems related to pregnancy. Most treat these ailments as a natural process and tend to ignore them, particularly, rural women who have had at least three to four children. Most women of higher parity face this problem more acutely. Hence, the respondents were asked questions on illness or any other problems they had encountered with their present or previous pregnancies.

Most women from Motipur, Kapgari, and Sultanpur did not complain of illness during pregnancy as compared to women from Santoshpur. Nearly (45%) of the women in Santhoshpur faced problems and illness during their pregnancy. In addition, the women from this village had the lowest number of antenatal care registration and check-ups (56%). For details see table 6.3.

Table 6.3:   **Per cent ill/sick during pregnancy**

VILLAGE	PROBLEMS DURING PREGNANCY (%)
MOTIPUR (Tribal, N_1 = 102)	6
KAPGARI (Hindu, N_2 = 100)	14
SANTOSHPUR (Muslim, N_3 = 100)	45
SULTANPUR (Developed, N_4 = 100)	12
TOTAL (N_T = 402)	77 (19.15%)

A large proportion of women from village Santoshpur had problems during pregnancy. This could be due to several and very close spaced pregnancies, lower age at marriage, child bearing at either very young or old ages. At the other extreme, only a negligible proportion of the tribal women in village Motipur complained of illness and problems during pregnancy. This could be attributed to the widespread self-neglect characteristic of many women, especially those women who also contribute to the household income. Such women tend to be inattentive to their own illness and health needs and fail to seek care.

The most common kind of complaint with pregnancy was that of dizziness, weakness and severe vomiting, closely followed by swelling of hands and legs and severe abdominal pain. Besides, there were a variety of complaints like epilepsy, acidity, lower backache and so on. However, a majority of the surveyed women sought treatment for their ailments. For details see table 6.4.

Table 6.4:   **Percentage sought treatment for ailment of those who experienced illness**

VILLAGE	(%) EXPERIENCED ILLNESS DURING PREGNANCY	PERCENT SOUGHT TREATMENT
MOTIPUR (Tribal, N_1 = 102)	6	6 (100%)
KAPGARI (Hindu, N_2 = 100)	14	12 (86%)
SANTOSHPUR (Muslim, N_3 = 100)	45	31 (69%)
SULTANPUR (Developed, N_4 = 100)	12	12 (100%)
TOTAL (N_T = 402)	77 (19.15%)	61 (15.17%)

It is interesting to note that almost all women who had encountered some sort of problems during pregnancy from the tribal village of Motipur and Sultanpur, sought immediate treatment for their ailments during pregnancy. In comparison, only 86 per cent women from village Kapgari, and 69 per cent from village Santoshpur (which incidentally had the highest number of complaints), sought treatment for their illness during pregnancy. This could probably be because of the widespread notion that illnesses and health problems are frequent during pregnancy and medical intervention is unnecessary.

The survey data also reveals the type of medical preference of the study population. The data reveals that the women of villages Motipur and Santoshpur, preferred the public sector for treatment. Whereas the women of villages Kapgari, and Sultanpur, relied heavily on the private medical sector for treatment. This preference can be explained by the fact that the women of the latter two villages are biased against the public medical sector and prefer the private medical sector. This is because the primary health centre in Kapgari is just a skeletal institution and the service delivery of the health centre is less than adequate. Therefore they are forced to use the private medical sector for treatment. Furthermore, the overall socio-economic condition and development of village Sultanpur is better than that of the other villages and they can afford to seek treatment from the private sector.

In addition, there is a common belief in the rural areas of India that most of the government hospitals/clinics, primary health centres are not good enough since the treatment and medicines are free. People in the study area did complain that since the medicines given from the PHCs were free, same medicines were prescribed always and given for all sorts of ailments. Therefore, economically better off people in the village, and, sometimes, even poor people take loans to visit the private medical sector for treatment. Refer to table 6.5 for details on kind of treatment for ailments sought during pregnancy.

Table 6. 5:   Kind of treatment sought for ailment during pregnancy

TREATMENT SOUGHT	MOTIPUR (Tribal, N_1 = 6)	KAPGARI (Hindu, N_2 = 12)	SANTOSHPUR (Muslim, N_3 = 31)	SULTANPUR (Developed, N_4 = 12)	TOTAL (N_T = 61)
PUBLIC SECTOR					
GOVT. HOSP.	1(16.66%)	2(16.66%)	-	5(41.66%)	8(13.11%)
PHC	3(50%)	2(16.66%)	20(64.51%)	-	25(40.98%)
SUB-CENTRE	-	1(8.33%)	-	-	1(1.63%)
PRIVATE MEDICAL SECTOR					
PRIVATE HOSPITAL/CLINIC	-	2(16.66%)	1(3.22%)	1(8.33%)	4(6.55%)
PHARMACY	-	-	1(3.22%)	-	1(1.63%)
PRIVATE DOCTOR	1(16.66%)	5(41.66%)	7(22.58%)	5(41.66%)	18(29.50%)
OTHER PRIVATE SECTOR					
HOMEOPATH DOCTOR	-	-	1 (3.22%)	1 (8.33%)	2 (3.27%)
OTHER SOURCE	1 (16.66%)	-	1 (3.22%)	-	2 (3.27%)
TOTAL	6 (9.83%)	12 (19.67%)	31 (50.81%)	12 (19.67%)	61

The women of village Santoshpur who did not seek any treatment for their illness during pregnancy were of the opinion that it was not essential and necessary at all. A majority of the women felt that illness and health problems were a natural part of pregnancy. The women said that after delivery everything would be normal, hence there was no need to worry about illness during pregnancy. A few women from village Kapgari also had similar views.

Overall three-fourths of the surveyed women had registered for antenatal care and check-ups. However, only one half of the surveyed women from the Muslim village of Santoshpur had registered for antenatal care, because they thought antenatal care was not essential as pregnancy is a natural process. Many women were also visited at home by health staff and health workers from the health centres and the government hospitals during their pregnancies.

Food Intake

In some societies many taboos and restrictions are imposed on women. These are generally imposed as a control mechanism in order to keep women in their 'place' in the social hierarchy. Taboos on women cover a wide perspective of things and range from controlling their movements, decision-making, status within the family, type of clothes they wear, food they consume during certain periods of their lives, and so on. India is one such society which imposes many restrictions on women, especially pregnant and lactating women, widows and unmarried girls, and girls who have attained puberty. These taboos and restrictions still hold true in the rural areas, particularly during pregnancy and lactation (Refer to chapter 2). Information was gathered on taboos practised during pregnancy and lactation. Restrictions during both these periods are placed on the kind and type of food a woman can consume, rituals to be observed and certain safety measures to be followed for safe delivery. In addition to food taboos, a number of other taboos and rituals are observed during this period.

> Sushila always had difficulty knowing when she was pregnant as she has irregular period, and whenever she is ill, her menstruation stops completely for a while. She was never very sure of her pregnancy until the 5th month. She was never very hungry during all her three pregnancies and did not feel like eating anything at all. She observed and followed the taboo and restrictions imposed on her during pregnancy and lactation as she lives in a joint household and can not disobey the elders. She was not allowed to go anywhere after dark, was not allowed to visit her natal home because of the fear that the journey could be fatal for the unborn child and the child could be harmed by evil spirits. She registered for an antenatal check-up for the first time during the 7th month of her pregnancy. In the 5th month of pregnancy prayers are offered to the family god and goddess along with the rest of the household, after which she was not allowed to eat eggs, onions, garlic, sea-food (like shells, clamps, crabs, prawns) certain types of fish, any kind of sour food, certain types of green leafy vegetables, papayas, egg-plants, pumpkins, gourds, etc.

The study found that a majority of the women from all villages except Sultanpur followed taboos and avoided certain kinds of food considered to be harmful both for the mother and the child. The food normally avoided during pregnancy are eggs, certain types of fish, milk, meat, certain kinds of vegetables like drumsticks, pumpkins, aubergines, papayas, and in some cases even potatoes. Certain green leafy vegetables which grow abundantly in the kitchen gardens of the households are also avoided.

The study indicates that the women of village Santoshpur did not include any sour foods in their diet when pregnant and avoided eating any kind of sea-food. These foods are believed to cause a number of problems during pregnancy and the child could be born with some defects. It is also believed that certain vegetables if eaten during pregnancy cause spontaneous abortion. The tragedy of food avoidance in the surveyed villages is that most households grow food the pregnant women are not supposed to eat.

Another taboo observed is that of restricted movement of pregnant mothers. They are not allowed to go anywhere after dark because of the fear of evil spirits, ghosts, supernatural beings, etc. They are further forbidden to wear any new clothes and jewellery. Moreover, they are not allowed to attend any funeral and are also not allowed to visit any new born babies. In addition to these a number of other taboos are observed in all the study villages.

Since West Bengal is a rice growing state, the staple diet of the population is rice. However, households with a higher level of income include a variety of vegetables, fish, meat and so on in their diet along with rice as opposed to households with low incomes. Most of the respondents stated rice to be their staple diet along with vegetables, lentils and pulses.

Normally my diet consists of tea and rice crisps in the morning, followed by leftover rice of the previous night which has been immersed in water in a heavy bottomed pan, with some vegetables. Sometimes, I do eat egg, fish and meat with this leftover rice. When I was pregnant I ate whatever I could afford. But most of the times I only had some green leafy vegetables and rice. Even during my pregnancy I had to first serve food to my husband and in-laws. I usually ate whatever was leftover after everybody in the household had finished eating. Sometimes the quantity of leftover food was not enough for me, but I never bothered to cook again only for myself as I was often very tired after attending to all the household chores and working in the fields. During all my pregnancies I felt very dizzy and weak. During my other two pregnancies, most of the times, I had nothing to eat at all because I am unable to support myself and my family on my meagre earnings. My husband was not with me during the other pregnancies and did not support me in any way during these pregnancies. He started living with another woman after our first child was born and he still lives with this woman and does not support us any longer. Though he visits us occasionally since he lives in the same village.

In village Santoshpur, 16 per cent reported that besides rice, vegetables and pulses, they regularly had either fish, meat or eggs, and milk, fruits etc. Similarly 20 per cent of the women from village Sultanpur stated that their daily diet consisted of rice, vegetables, lentils, either fish, meat or eggs, fruits and milk.

Nearly two-thirds of the women stated that their quantity of food intake was similar to that of the other members of the household during normal times and even during pregnancy. However, a large proportion of the women did not increase their diet during pregnancy. Only a third of the pregnant women had ever increased their food intake during pregnancy. Refer to table 6.6. for more details.

Table 6.6:   **Food intake during pregnancy**

VILLAGE	QUANTITY OF FOOD INTAKE SIMILAR TO OTHER MEMBERS OF THE HOUSEHOLD	INCREASED FOOD INTAKE DURING PREGNANCY
MOTIPUR (Tribal, $N_1 = 102$)	60	15
KAPGARI (Hindu, $N_2 = 100$)	64	31
SANTOSHPUR (Muslim, $N_3 = 100$)	63	45
SULTANPUR (Developed, $N_4 = 100$)	84	31
TOTAL ($N_T = 402$)	271 (67.41%)	122 (30.34%)

The table indicates that very few women in Motipur had increased their food intake during pregnancy. This is because the economic condition of a majority of the households surveyed in this village is below the poverty level. Many women live in joint families where preference in terms of food distribution and consumption is given to the male members and children. Pregnant women usually eat the leftovers which is not always enough both in quantity and quality. The women in Santoshpur could afford to increase their diet during pregnancy because of their comparative better socio-economic status than the villagers of Motipur. Furthermore, a majority of the surveyed households were nuclear and the women could make decisions regarding food distribution, allocation and consumption patterns within the family .

Many surveyed respondents consumed some sort of special foods during pregnancy. The most preferred common food for pregnant women in Motipur is a preparation made from various pulses and lentils with sugar. Sixteen per cent of the women in Motipur consumed this special preparation and some even had milk and fruits. In Kapgari 22 per cent had milk, eggs, fruits, special types of fish, and certain types of green vegetables supposed to be good for the health of the mother and the baby during pregnancy.

Despite the taboos and restrictions on food for pregnant women, more than half of the women in Santoshpur ate meat, fish, eggs, milk, fruits, etc. during pregnancy. Twenty-one per cent of the women in Sultanpur included fruits, milk, eggs, meat etc. in their diet during pregnancy. Some of the pregnant women in Sultanpur were also supplied with supplementary nutrition through the Anganwadi Centre.

Poverty was cited as a major problem for not increasing food intake during pregnancy. In village Motipur, 63 per cent said they were too poor to eat properly, and to consume special foods during pregnancy or for that matter increase their daily food intake. Similar responses were given by 40 per cent of the women in Kapgari, 30 per cent in village Santoshpur and 22 per cent in village Sultanpur.

Workload

Women in general undertake a disproportionately greater share of total household work, that is, economic work and household domestic work combined. Women in India also work longer hours in paid plus unpaid/domestic work than men. Women undertake arduous tasks such as fetching water, collecting fuel and fodder, tending cattle, cooking, washing and cleaning the house, washing clothes, utensils, caring for children and the sick, and so on, from a very early age.

The surveyed women also undertook all the domestic chores, in addition to agricultural work. The normal working day for rural women in India begins with the sun-rise and ends when they go to bed after catering to their family's wants and needs, which very often is as late as 11 p.m. Normal working day duties include fetching water, firewood, feeding cattle, cleaning cattle-sheds, milking, cooking meals, cleaning the house, collecting cow-dung for fuel, washing clothes, utensils, feeding and caring for children, looking after the sick and any number of other household chores like husking and threshing of grains, etc. Moreover, they work as agricultural labourers during harvesting and sowing seasons and also help their spouses and children in the paddy fields. Furthermore, they prepare puffed rice and rice crisps for home consumption and also for selling in the market.

Normally I do all the household chores and I also help my husband in the fields during the sowing and harvesting seasons, and whenever he needs any help with his work in the fields. During all my pregnancies I continued doing all the usual chores. I generally get up at around five in the morning and start the day with sweeping and cleaning the house. Next I clean the cattle-shed and collect cow-dung for coating the yard and also to make cow-dung cakes for fuel for cooking. Then, I fetch water from the well for cooking and drinking. After all this I have a cup of tea and some rice-crisps. By then other members of the family wake up. I serve them tea and rice-crisps and then start cooking food. After all the men have eaten rice and some vegetables and lentils and left for work, I take all the dirty utensils, dishes and clothes for washing to the village pond. After this I again go to the village well to fetch water. I usually need to fetch water three times daily. By the time I finish all these chores it is usually 11. After this I have to bathe and feed the children and the elderly people of the household. Normally I husk and thresh the grain or prepare rice-crisps (*Muri*), or sew and repair old clothes or make blankets, quilts, knit, etc. By 12:30 p.m. I go for my bath to the village pond and after that eat whatever is leftover from the mornings cooking. During the afternoons I normally look after my children, or the older relatives in the household and tend to their needs, feed the cattle, fetch water again, and overall tend to other needs like gathering firewood, making fuel etc. By 4 p.m. I start making preparation for evening food and start cooking again. By 6 p.m. the men are back, I serve them tea and *Muri,* feed the children the same snack and go to the village pond with the dirty dishes and clothes. I have my bath again at this time. By 8 p.m. I start serving food to the men and children first, then the elderly members of the household, then the other members (womenfolk) of the house eat. After this I wash the kitchen, wash the verandah where we eat. Next I feed the cattle, secure all the gates, doors and windows of the house and put the children to bed. After this I have to tend to the needs of the elderly of the house, if they need anything or massaging them and also tend to my husbands needs. By the time I go to bed it is normally 11 p.m.

The study found an overwhelming percentage (92%) of the surveyed women continued with similar amount of workload during pregnancy even at advanced stages which they performed during normal times. The women who stopped doing their usual work during pregnancy said their doctors had advised full bed rest. Others said they were too weak and very dizzy to continue doing the same work properly and a few also complained of swollen hands and legs accompanied with intense pain which forced them to stop doing the usual chores. Furthermore, a few women were of the opinion that too much physical exertion would harm the baby hence they reduced their regular workload. Six per cent of the women from Sultanpur said they were too big during the last trimester of pregnancy and had difficulty in bending and doing the same amount of work.

A number of taboos and safety measures are observed and followed during pregnancy for a safe delivery. The study reveals that a majority of the surveyed women from all villages except Sultanpur followed the prescribed taboos in order to have a healthy baby and a safe delivery. Though two-thirds of the women claimed their quantity of food intake was similar to that of the other members of the household during normal times and even during pregnancy, the study indicates that an overwhelming majority did not increase their food intake during pregnancy. Poverty was cited as a major problem for not increasing food intake. Nearly all women continued with the same amount of workload both within and outside home during pregnancy and even at advanced stages when it becomes awfully difficult to do tedious and laborious work.

Labour and Delivery

In most of the developing societies women prefer home deliveries to institutional deliveries, despite attending antenatal clinics. Women at this time prefer to be surrounded by family members, relatives and friends. Other factors such as the prevalence of more male doctors in most of the health centres also discourage women from utilising the available health care facilities for labour and delivery. In many cultures a woman will not be allowed by her family and the community to be examined or attended by a male doctor. Moreover, the health staff at the health centres are also not considerate and tolerant towards illiterate women and are often uncourteous to the visiting family members and relatives. The women also feel intimidated by the health staff and doctors and can not voice their fear and concerns about childbirth and other related consequences of delivery. Because of these factors women prefer home deliveries, and feel childbirth to be a happy and joyful occasion, to be shared with family and friends.

> I delivered my youngest child at the village PHC. At the onset of my labour pains I was taken to the village PHC, as I had difficulties with my earlier deliveries at home. However, there were no doctors or nurses (no health

personnel were present at the PHC during my delivery) present to assist with my labour and delivery. Eventually the village *dai* was summoned to deliver my baby and to cut the umbilical cord at the PHC. I and my family members absolutely depend on the *dai* for everything, as most of the times there are no health personnel available in the village PHC to attend to labour and delivery. Therefore even during complications of delivery we depend on the village *dai* to take care of everything. If by any chance the delivery gets complicated and the *dai* is unable to handle it, it is pointless to take the patient to the district government hospital, because the doctors and the other health staff get angry with us for not coming to the hospital during the onset of labour pains and scold us and blame us for everything going wrong. I think it is useless to worry if the delivery gets complicated because we can't get any help from either the village PHC as health professionals are seldom available, or from the government hospitals where we are treated with disdain. Ultimately either the mother or the child might die with the complication of a delivery and this is a very natural process of childbirth and we have to endure it as we are women and we are born to endure all the hardships in life.

The survey data shows that the women in Motipur and Santoshpur had more home deliveries. The women of villages Kapgari and Sultanpur had a higher number of institutionalised deliveries. Refer to Table No. 6.7 for more information.

Table 6.7:   **Location of labour and delivery**

LABOUR & DELIVERY	MOTIPUR (Tribal, N_1 = 98)	KAPGARI (Hindu, N_2 = 98)	SANTOSHPUR (Muslim, N_3 = 92)	SULTANPUR (Developed, N_4 = 94)	TOTAL (N_T = 382)
HUSBAND'S HOME	85 (86.73%)	45 (45.91%)	45 (48.91%)	21 (22.34%)	196 (51.30%)
NATAL HOME	4 (4.08%)	3 (3.06%)	25 (27.17%)	5 (5.31%)	37 (9.68%)
OTHER PLACE	-	-	-	1 (1.06%)	1 (0.26%)
GOVT. /MUNICIPAL HOSP.	2 (2.04%)	10 (10.20%)	3 (3.26%)	59 (62.76%)	74 (19.37%)
PHC	7 (7.14%)	32 (32.65%)	19 (20.65%)	2 (2.12%)	60 (15.70%)
SUB-CENTRE	-	3 (3.06%)	-	-	3 (0.78%)
PRIVATE HOSP. /CLINIC	-	5 (5.10%)	-	6 (6.38%)	11 (2.87%)
TOTAL	98	98	92	94	382

The data shows that women in village Motipur prefer home deliveries as opposed to institutional deliveries. This is because they do not trust any strangers and most of all the health and the community workers. They regard any strangers as family planning workers. Moreover, their experience during the 'Emergency Period' (1975-77), when many people, especially the poor and illiterate villagers were forcibly sterilised. Therefore the poor and illiterate villagers of Motipur look upon any strangers or health care officials with suspicion and are wary of institutionalised deliveries, as they reckon sterilisation could be performed immediately after childbirth without their knowledge or consent. The table further indicates that the women in Santoshpur also favour home deliveries.

However, both the villages of Kapgari and Sultanpur had more institutionalised deliveries. This can be attributed to more years spent in school for both the men and the women of the two villages. In addition, both the villages are socially more developed and the villagers are aware of the available health care facilities. Furthermore, the primary occupation of a majority of the villagers in Sultanpur is not related to farming and most of them work in the district town and the city. Kapgari has research institutions and schools and a college in the village which contributes towards knowledge and awareness.

The data further reveals that most of the deliveries in Motipur was conducted by non-professionals, a majority of them by relatives and friends. In Santoshpur too, more than one half of the deliveries were conducted by the Traditional Birth Attendants (TBA), called '*dai*'. In Kapgari 52 per cent of the deliveries were handled by professionals and 74 per cent in Sultanpur were assisted by health professionals. Refer to table 6.8.

Table 6.8:   **Type of assistance with delivery**

ASSISTANCE AT DELIVERY	MOTIPUR (Tribal, N_1 = 98)	KAPGARI (Hindu, N_2 = 98)	SANTOSHPUR Muslim, N_3 = 92)	SULTANPUR (Developed, N_4 = 94)	TOTAL (N_T = 382)
HEALTH PROFESSIONALS					
DOCTORS	2 (2.04%)	20 (20.40%)	5 (5.43%)	17 (18.08%)	44 (11.51%)
AYURVEDIC DOC./VAID	2 (2.04%)	-	2 (2.17%)	1 (1.06%)	5 (1.30%)
NURSE/MIDWIFE	8 (8.16%)	27 (27.55%)	15 (16.30%)	46 (48.93%)	96 (25.13%)
ANM/LHV	-	5 (5.10%)	-	-	5 (1.30%)
OTHER PERSONS					
TRAINED TBA	-	-	12 (13.04%)	10 (10.63%)	22 (5.75%)
TBA/DAI	3 (3.06%)	4 (4.08%)	56 (60.86%)	16 (17.02%)	79 (20.68%)
RELATIVES/FRIENDS	65 (66.32%)	34 (34.69%)	2 (2.17%)	2 (2.12%)	103 (26.96%)
OTHER	18 (18.36%)	8 (8.16%)	-	2 (2.12%)	28 (7.32%)
TOTAL	98	98	92	94	382

The table shows that only 12 per cent of the deliveries in Motipur were handled by health professionals as opposed to 88 per cent handled by other persons. In village Santoshpur, about a quarter (23.9%) of the deliveries were assisted by health professionals, and the rest (76.1%) by other persons. This is because the women do not like to be attended to by male doctors.

In Kapgari more than half (53%) the deliveries were handled by trained health professionals, and in Sultanpur 68 per cent were conducted by health professionals. This can be explained because of higher literacy, socio-economic status and awareness of modern health care services in both the villages.

Normally pregnant women are admitted to any medical establishment with the onset of labour pains, but this is not true for most cases in the study villages. In Motipur, assistance was sought only after delivery. The *dai* was specifically called to cut the umbilical cord and to clean the mother and the child. This was true in two-thirds of the cases. In Kapgari 28 per cent sought help after delivery while in Santoshpur 10 per cent called for assistance after delivery, and 5 per cent did the same in Sultanpur. See table 6.9 for more information.

Table 6.9: **When assistance was sought for labour and delivery**

VILLAGE	AFTER DELIVERY	DURING INTENSE PAIN	WHEN WATER BROKE	TOTAL
MOTIPUR (Tribal, N_1 = 98)	65 (66.32%)	28 (28.57%)	5 (5.10%)	98
KAPGARI (Hindu, N_2 = 98)	28 (28.57%)	57 (58.16%)	13 (13.26%)	98
SANTOSHPUR (Muslim, N_3 = 92)	10 (10.86%)	71 (77.17)	11 (11.95%)	92
SULTANPUR (Developed, N_4 = 94)	5 (5.31%)	77 (81.91%)	12 (12.76%)	94
TOTAL (N_T = 382)	108 (28.27%)	233 (60.99%)	41 (10.73%)	382

The data reveals that with the exception of Motipur, women in the other study villages had received assistance at the onset of labour pains. In Kapgari more than half had either called for assistance or taken the patient to the nearest health centre. Whereas in Santoshpur and Sultanpur a majority had sought assistance after the onset of labour pains. The women in Motipur said that since they did not face any problems with their delivery they did not call for any assistance.

Even though women in Motipur had a maximum number of home deliveries, only eight per cent said they encountered any problems during delivery. This may be because the women feel that complications are a natural part of delivery and do not report such occurrence. In Kapgari, 16 per cent faced complications. More than a third of the women in Santoshpur had problems delivering their last child. The women in Santoshpur had 4-6 children (see family size and composition, in Chapter 3), and pregnancy, labour and delivery at an advanced age becomes complicated due to the depleted nutritional status of the mother. See table 6.10.

Table 6.10:   **Complications faced during delivery**

VILLAGE	COMPLICATIONS FACED DURING DELIVERY
MOTIPUR (Tribal, N_1 = 98)	8 (8.16%)
KAPGARI (Hindu, N_2 = 98)	16 (16.32%)
SANTOSHPUR (Muslim, N_3 = 92)	39 (42.39%)
SULTANPUR (Developed, N_4 = 94)	13 (13.82%)
TOTAL (N_T = 382)	76 (19.89%)

The most common type of complication during delivery (faced by almost a third of the women) is that of a long period of labour, sometimes more than 24 hours or more. The next common complaint was that of excessive bleeding during delivery, followed by delayed delivery of the placenta, and so on. See table 6.11.

Table 6.11:   **Kind of complications faced during delivery**

KIND OF COMPLICATIONS	MOTIPUR (Tribal, N_1 = 8)	KAPGARI (Hindu, N_2 = 16)	SANTOSHPUR (Muslim, N_3 = 39)	SULTANPUR (Developed, N_4 = 13)	TOTAL (N_T = 76)
LONG PERIOD OF LABOUR	5 (62.5%)	4 (25%)	23 (58.97%)	1 (7.69%)	33 (43.42%)
DELAYED DELIVERY OF PLACENTA	3 (37.5%)	1 (6.25%)	3 (7.69%)	1 (7.69%)	8 (10.52%)
EXCESSIVE BLEEDING	-	6 (37.5%)	10 (25.64%)	-	16 (21.05%)
CESAREAN SECTION	-	2 (12.5%)	2 (5.12%)	3 (23.07%)	7 (9.21%)
USE OF FORCEPS	-	-	1 (2.56%)	1 (7.69%)	2 (2.63%)
OTHER	-	3 (18.75%)	-	7 (53.84%)	10 (13.15%)
TOTAL	8 (10.52%)	16 (21.05%)	39 (51.31%)	13 (17.10%)	76

Almost 59 per cent of the women in Santoshpur had a long period of labour and a quarter encountered excessive bleeding during delivery. This is mainly due to either chronic under-nutrition and/or malnutrition of the mothers, anaemia, low-weight gain during pregnancy, small pelvis, or delivery at an early age (13-18 years of age) or at an advanced age (39-49 years) of the mother. In Kapgari too, 38 per cent of the women had excessive bleeding and a quarter experienced a long period of labour. Whilst in Motipur 63 per cent experienced a long period of labour and 37 per cent had complications due to delayed delivery of the placenta. All these problems and complications during labour and delivery are the result of either age of the mother, parity, birth order of the child, nutritional status of the mother and/or other socio-economic factors.

In the case of home deliveries, when complications arise related to delivery or labour, the women in Motipur depend almost entirely on the *dai* to take care of problems in 97 per cent of the cases. Only three per cent prefer to take the patient to the nearest government hospital. The women do not utilise the services of the village PHC because of fear and depend entirely on *dai's* even during an emergency.

The PHC in Kapgari is just a skeletal structure. A nurse runs the centre in the mornings from 7 AM until 10:30 AM, and the doctor is never available, as he lives in Calcutta. Therefore the villagers hardly ever utilise the services of the health centre. In Kapgari, 63 per cent relied entirely on the *dai*; 33 per cent preferred the village PHC in case of complications and another 4 per cent rushed the patient to the nearest government hospital for treatment.

Though the PHC in Santoshpur is well staffed with a 30-bed capacity, and the four doctors and all the nurses are always on duty and on call 24 hours a day, a large number of deliveries were conducted at home. Sixty-six per cent of the women preferred the village PHC to treat any complications arising due to labour and delivery, whereas 11 per cent straight away took the patient to the nearest government hospital and the remaining 23 per cent relied absolutely on the *dai* to take care of everything. More women utilise the services of the village PHC because of its easy accessibility and availability of the health staff during emergencies and complications.

In Sultanpur, only seven per cent relied on the *dai* in case of complications, 18 per cent took the patient to the village PHC and seven per cent called a doctor or a nurse at home for treatment, 67 per cent took the patient to the nearest government hospital. The people of this village did not entirely rely on the services of the village PHC because the district government hospital is near by and because of easy communication and transportation facilities prefer the government hospital for treatment as there are more doctors, more beds and more modern amenities to deal with complications and other problems arising due to labour and delivery. Though the PHC is well staffed and has a 15-bed capacity very few people utilise its services. Refer to table 6.12.

Table 6.12:   **Kind of help sought due to complication of delivery**

HELP SOUGHT DUE TO COMPLICATIONS OF DELIVERY	MOTIPUR (Tribal, N_1 = 89)	KAPGARI (Hindu, N_2 = 48)	SANTOSHPUR (Muslim, N_3 = 70)	SULTANPUR (Developed, N_4 = 27)	TOTAL (N_T = 234)
No. OF HOME DELIVERIES	**89**	**48**	**70**	**27**	**234**
DEPEND ON DAI/TBA	86 (96.62%)	30 (62.5%)	16 (22.85%)	2 (7.40%)	134 (57.26%)
VILLAGE PHC	-	16 (33.33%)	46 (65.71%)	5 (18.51%)	67 (28.63%)
GOVERNMENT HOSPITAL	3 (3.37%)	2 (4.16%)	8 (11.42%)	18 (66.66%)	31 (13.24%)
CALL DOCTOR/NURSE AT HOME	-	-	-	2 (7.40%)	2 (0.85%)
TOTAL	89 (38.03%)	48 (20.51%)	70 (29.91%)	27 (11.53%)	234

The extreme dependence on *dai* could be either due to ignorance, illiteracy, lack of knowledge of services, lack of communication or transportation, or just a feeling of apprehension towards health centres and health personnel. Besides, health personnel are seldom available at the health centres to attend to emergencies.

In case of home deliveries most of the times sterilised razor blades were used to cut the umbilical cord. In very few cases other instruments such as bamboo blades, kitchen knives, scissors, used blades, were used to cut the cord. See table 6.13.

Table 6.13:   Instrument used to cut the umbilical cord

INSTRUMENT USED TO CUT UMBILICAL CORD	MOTIPUR (Tribal, N_1 = 98)	KAPGARI (Hindu, N_2 = 98)	SANTOSHPUR (Muslim, N_3 = 92)	SULTANPUR (Developed, N_4 = 94)	TOTAL (N_T = 382)
STERILISED SCISSORS	10 (10.20%)	51 (52.04%)	27 (29.34%)	28 (29.78%)	116 (30.36%)
STERILISED RAZOR BLADES	78 (79.59%)	43 (43.87%)	56 (60.86%)	55 (58.51%)	232 (60.73%)
USED BLADES	1 (1.02%)	2 (2.04%)	1 (1.08%)	1 (1.06%)	5 (1.30%)
BAMBOO BLADES	5 (5.10%)	-	2 (2.17%)	1 (1.06%)	8 (2.09%)
SCISSORS	-	1 (1.02%)	-	-	1 (0.26%)
KITCHEN KNIVES	-	-	1 (1.08%)	-	1 (0.26%)
OTHER	4 (4.08%)	1 (1.02%)	5 (5.43%)	9 (9.57%)	19 (4.97%)
TOTAL	98	98	92	94	382

In Kapgari more than one half used sterilised scissors to cut the cord. This is because the health centre distributes sterilised delivery kit to the *dais* in Kapgari. Even though a majority of the deliveries in Sultanpur was conducted at health centres and hospitals, only 30 per cent reported that sterilised scissors had been used to cut the cord. This is either due to erroneous recording, or the women themselves were unaware of the instruments used to cut the cord. A majority of the women who delivered at home said, the cord stump was closed by placing old, clean rags or cotton wool with medication, normally dettol. It was then tied up with sewing thread. In some cases the stump was tied with a thread without any medication.

Most of the women said, their placenta was delivered almost immediately after delivery. In a third of the cases, the placenta was delivered after half an hour, and in 12 per cent after an hour or so, and in 3 per cent it was delayed for more than two hours or more. See table 6.14 for details.

Table 6.14:   Delivery of placenta

VILLAGE	IMMEDIATELY	AFTER 30 MINUTES	AN HOUR LATER	AFTER TWO OR MORE HOURS	TOTAL
MOTIPUR (Tribal, N_1 = 98)	89 (90.81%)	4 (4.08%)	5 (5.10%)	-	98
KAPGARI (Hindu, N_2 = 98)	97 (98.97%)	-	1 (1.02%)	-	98
SANTOSHPUR (Muslim, N_3 = 92)	62 (67.39%)	23 (25%)	4 (4.34%)	3 (3.26%)	92
SULTANPUR (Developed, N_4 = 94)	89 (94.68%)	3 (3.19%)	2 (2.12%)	-	94
TOTAL (N_T = 382)	337 (88.21%)	30 (7.85%)	12 (3.14%)	3 (0.78%)	382

The table indicates that 88 per cent of the women immediately delivered the placenta after delivery. But for a quarter of the women in Santoshpur, delivering the placenta took more than half an hour after child birth. The delayed delivery of placenta could either be due to an abnormality in the uterus or due to maternal exhaustion because of long period of labour. Additionally, sometimes the placenta adheres to the uterine walls in an abnormal way, which can lead to the delayed delivery of placenta. Problems such as infection (septicaemia) of the uterus, or infertility, are caused by a retained placenta leading to either illness or death of the mother.

My last child was delivered at home by relatives and they did not think it was necessary to call the *dai* so late at night as I delivered at 02:00 A.M. The *dai* was sent for in the morning to cut the umbilical cord and to clean me and my baby. The cord was cut with a sterilised blade and the stump was closed with a sewing thread. My placenta too delivered itself after the baby was born. The *dai* placed the placenta in an earthen-ware pitcher and covered it with a lid and buried it in the ground within the room where I had delivered. It is a tradition to bury the placenta so that the new-born or the mother does not fall prey to the evil spirits immediately after birth, as this is the time when we are most susceptible for possession by evil forces. I underwent a sterilisation when my youngest born was 12 days old as I did not want any more children. I was on the pills for a while but often I forgot to take them and eventually became pregnant.

In most developing societies women prefer to have home deliveries and this was found to be true in the study population as well. More than one half of the women had deliveries at home conducted by either friends or relatives or by *dais*. A majority of the women in Motipur and Santoshpur had home deliveries as opposed to the women from Kapgari and Sultanpur. Most of the women sought assistance and help at the onset of intense labour pains, while a large number of women in Motipur sought help and assistance only after delivery. A majority of the women in Santoshpur faced complications with the delivery of their last child. The most common problem was that of long period of labour and excessive bleeding. In case of home deliveries, sterilised razor blades were used to cut the umbilical cord in most cases. A large proportion of women delivering at home, delivered the placenta immediately after child birth.

Two of my older children were delivered at my natal home by my family members and friends as the *dai* arrived late. The youngest was born at the village PHC. During my first delivery, my mother sent somebody to bring the *dai* at the onset of my labour pains. Since the *dai* lives in another village, far away from my mother's house, She arrived late. By then I had already given birth to a baby girl. The *dai* arrived after an hour. I was still lying on the mud floor where I had given birth with the baby attached to the umbilical cord in a pool of blood. None of my family members attended to me or made an attempt to move me or clean me. The *dai* on her arrival finally cut the umbilical cord with a blade provided by my mother which was sterilised in boiling water and cleaned me and the baby with the help of old rags provided by my mother. I did not face any difficulty with the delivery of my first child and even the placenta delivered itself without any problems.

Postnatal Care and Check-ups

After childbirth and delivery, many times women suffer from health related problems. The same has been found in the study population. Although, the degree and level of problems varied between villages, some of the complaints were very similar in almost all of the study villages.

In Motipur only 9 per cent of the women reported that they had encountered health problems after delivery. This low level of reporting is due to a high level of pain tolerance and discomfort by these women. Only 7 per cent in Kapgari said they ever faced any health problems after the delivery of their last child. Overall, 17 per cent had health problems after delivery. See table 6.15 for more details.

Table 6.15:   Health problems after delivery

VILLAGE	HEALTH PROBLEMS AFTER DELIVERY	TOTAL
MOTIPUR (Tribal, N_1 = 98)	9 (9.18%)	98
KAPGARI (Hindu, N_2 = 98)	7 (7.14%)	98
SANTOSHPUR (Muslim, N_3 = 92)	38 (41.30%)	92
SULTANPUR (Developed, N_4 = 94)	12 (12.76%)	94
TOTAL (N_T = 382)	66 (17.27%)	382

The table points that 41 per cent of the women in Santoshpur faced health problems after delivery (a higher number of women in this village had problems/illness during pregnancy as well). This could be because of the number of children they had borne either at an advanced age or at an early age, and also close spaced pregnancies, whereby the mother does not get a chance to recover and build up her nutritional resources, physical strength and energy. In Sultanpur 13 per cent of the women reportedly suffered from health problems after the delivery of their last child.

Table 6.16 gives information on types of health problems encountered by women after delivery. The data shows that nearly 70 per cent of the women suffered from severe weakness, giddiness, dizziness and symptoms of feeling faint.

Table 6.16   Types of health problem after delivery

KINDS/TYPES OF HEALTH PROBLEMS	MOTIPUR (Tribal, N_1 = 9)	KAPGARI (Hindu, N_2 = 7)	SANTOSHPUR (Muslim, N_3 = 38)	SULTANPUR (Developed, N_4 = 12)	TOTAL (N_T = 66)
SEVERE WEAKNESS, DIZZINESS, ETC.	8 (88.88%)	4 (57.14%)	28 (73.68%)	6 (50%)	46 (69.69%)
HIGH FEVER	-	1 (14.28%)	4 (10.52%)	-	5 (7.57%)
BLOOD CLOT IN THE UTERUS	-	1 (14.28%)	-	-	1 (1.51%)
PAIN IN THE STITCHES & SUTURES	-	1 (14.28%)	-	4 (33.33%)	5 (7.57%)
ASTHMA	1 (11.11%)	-	-	-	1 (1.51%)
HIGH BLOOD PRESSURE	-	-	1 (2.63%)	-	1 (1.51%)
PILES	-	-	1 (2.63%)	-	1 (1.51%)
SEVERE ACIDITY	-	-	3 (7.89%)	-	3 (4.54%)
SWOLLEN HANDS & LEGS	-	-	1 (2.63%)	1 (8.33%)	2 (3.03%)
UNDERWENT STERILIZATION	-	-	-	1 (8.33%)	1 (1.51%)
TOTAL WOMEN (HEALTH PROBLEMS)	9	7	38	12	66

The symptoms can be explained because of chronic under-nutrition or malnutrition, anaemia during pregnancy, and probably through out their entire life, followed by early marriage, early childbearing and rearing, along with strenuous and laborious working hours, breast feeding and other related factors associated with the health of mother. Refer to the table for more details on health problems after delivery.

Bouts of severe weakness, dizziness, giddiness are also because of the quality and quantity of food intake of the women during pregnancy. Furthermore, after delivery women follow certain rituals and taboos to purify them and to remove the polluting effects. They are not allowed to eat two meals a day, and are allowed to eat only certain types of food during the first few days immediately after childbirth. This makes them weaker immediately after child birth. This high percentage of complaints about weakness can be explained by the chronic under-nutrition and malnutrition of the women in their childhood years, as well as later, and especially during pregnancies. Malnutrition during pregnancy inevitably leads to anaemia and other related problems like long period of labour, excessive bleeding during delivery and delayed delivery of placenta, which in turn leads to poor lactation.

The women in villages Motipur and Sultanpur who faced health problems after delivery sought some kind of treatment and medical attention. But, in villages Kapgari and Santoshpur a quarter of the women with problems did not seek any medical attention. Refer to table 6.17 for more details.

Table 6.17:   Type of treatment sought for problems after delivery

TREATMENT AFTER DELIVERY	MOTIPUR (Tribal, $N_1 = 9$)	KAPGARI (Hindu, $N_2 = 7$)	SANTOSHPUR (Muslim, $N_3 = 38$)	SULTANPUR (Developed, $N_4 = 12$)	TOTAL ($N_T = 66$)
PUBLIC SECTOR					
GOVT./MUNICIPAL HOSP.	-	1 (14.28%)	1 (2.63%)	7 (58.33%)	9 (13.63%)
PHC	6 (66.66%)	1 (14.28%)	19 (50%)	1 (8.33%)	27 (40.90%)
SUB-CENTRE	-	-	-	1 (8.33%)	1 (1.51%)
PRIVATE SECTOR					
PRIVATE HOSP./CLINIC	-	1 (14.28%)	-	-	1 (1.51%)
PRIVATE DOCTOR	2 (22.22%)	1 (14.28%)	2 (5.26%)	3 (25%)	8 (12.12%)
OTHER PRIVATE SECTOR					
SHOP	-	-	1 (2.63%)	-	1 (1.51%)
TRADITIONAL PRACTITIONER	-	1 (14.28%)	1 (2.63%)	-	2 (3.03%)
HOMEOPATH DOCTOR	-	-	4 (10.52%)	-	4 (6.06%)
OTHER	1 (11.11%)	-	1 (2.63%)	-	2 (3.03%)
TOTAL	9 (100%)	5 (71.42%)	29 (76.31%)	12 (100%)	55 (83.33%)

In Kapgari 29 per cent of the women did not seek any treatment for their illness after delivery. Likewise, 24 per cent of the women in Santoshpur did not seek any medical attention for their health problems. Most of the women in Santoshpur who did not bother to seek any medical attention for their health problems after delivery thought illness and health problems to be a natural part of the child bearing process. A few reported that they were not allowed to go for treatment or they did not have the time. Financial constraint was also cited by some women as the reason for not seeking treatment. The women in Kapgari also thought it was not necessary to pursue treatment for health problems after delivery because it was inconvenient to visit health centres in view of their seclusion after delivery. As a result of these restrictions, customs, norms, values, and mores, very few women attended a postnatal clinic. Refer to table 6.18 for more details.

Table 6.18:   Percentage going for a postnatal check-up

VILLAGE	WENT FOR A POSTNATAL CHECKUP YES	NO	TOTAL
MOTIPUR (Tribal, $N_1 = 98$)	20 (20.40%)	78 (79.59%)	98
KAPGARI (Hindu, $N_2 = 98$)	38 (38.77%)	60 (61.22%)	98
SANTOSHPUR (Muslim, $N_3 = 92$)	37 (40.21%)	55 (59.78%)	92
SULTANPUR (Developed, $N_4 = 94$)	32 (34.04%)	62 (65.95%)	94
TOTAL ($N_T = 382$)	127 (33.24%)	255 (66.75%)	382

Overall a third of the women went for a postnatal check-up. This low percentage of postnatal clinic attendance is due to the compulsory isolation and seclusion of the women and the new-born from everything for a certain period of time, or because of lack of knowledge and awareness about postnatal clinics and check-ups.

An overwhelming majority of the women thought it was unnecessary to attend a postnatal clinic, while others said, they were not aware of the utility of a postnatal clinic. According to a few it was not customary for them to attend postnatal clinics. See table 6.19 for more details on reasons for not attending postnatal clinics.

Table 6.19:   **Reasons for not attending postnatal clinics**

REASONS FOR NOT ATTENDING POSTNATAL CLINIC	MOTIPUR (Tribal, N_1 = 78)	KAPGARI (Hindu, N_2 = 60)	SANTOSHPUR (Muslim, N_3 = 55)	SULTANPUR (Developed, N_4 = 62)	TOTAL (N_T = 255)
NOT CUSTOMARY	3 (3.84%)	2 (3.33%)	4 (7.27%)	1 (1.61%)	10 (3.92%)
NOT NECESSARY	67 (85.89%)	55 (91.66%)	36 (65.45%)	51 (82.25%)	209 (81.96%)
LACK OF KNOWLEDGE	8 (10.25%)	2 (3.33%)	8 (14.54%)	10 (16.12%)	28 (10.98%)
FINANCIAL CONSTRAINT	-	-	3 (5.45%)	-	3 (1.17%)
INCONVENIENT	-	1 (1.66%)	-	-	1 (0.39%)
NO TIME TO GO	-	-	3 (5.45%)	-	3 (1.17%)
OTHER	-	-	1 (1.81%)	-	1 (0.39%)
TOTAL	78	60	55	62	255

Nearly 82 per cent of the women felt that postnatal clinic attendance was not necessary, and 11 per cent were not aware of the utility of postnatal clinics. The low level of utilisation of postnatal services can be explained by the fact that postnatal health care has not been widely publicised in the country, and that even the health centres and health personnel do not emphasise the need for such care. Hence, there is a wide spread ignorance about the subject and therefore, women think it is not essential or necessary to attend postnatal clinics. Furthermore, the older women in the villages never attended these clinics and never faced any problems by not attending such clinics. Consequently, the whole idea of attending a postnatal clinic seems ridiculous and unnecessary to the women of the study villages. Only those women who encountered health problems after childbirth went for a postnatal check-up and attended the postnatal clinics regularly.

The respondents who had delivered very recently (during the time of the survey) were not very sure if they would attend any postnatal clinics. A large number of women said it was not necessary, and they would not attend the clinics. But, if there were any health problems, then they would.

It seems there is a need to publicise and actively campaign more about postnatal health care, its benefits and importance in the rural areas of the country on a much wider scale to make women aware of the advantages of a postnatal check-up both for the mother and the child, or deploy female health staff to visit homes of the new-born to offer postnatal care, in view of the seclusion practised by most women because of their belief in pollution after childbirth (discussed in the following chapter).

Conclusion

The study found that a majority of the surveyed women had registered for antenatal care during their previous and/or current pregnancies. The most number of complaints regarding illness during pregnancy were found in the Muslim village, and the women in this village had the lowest number of antenatal registrations. Food taboos were religiously observed in the study villages during pregnancy, except in the developed village. Very few surveyed women increased their food intake during pregnancy. Poverty was cited as a major hindrance in increasing the quantity of food intake. An overwhelming percentage of the women continued with the same amount of tedious and laborious workload during pregnancy. Most of the deliveries in Motipur and Santoshpur were conducted at home assisted by *dais* as opposed to the other two study villages, where most of the births were institutionalised. Sterilised razor blades were used to cut the umbilical cord in home deliveries. Postnatal care is found to be minimal because of lack of awareness and knowledge regarding postnatal services and its benefits and also because of the belief that it is not essential and/or necessary.

Cultural Practices and Postnatal Care

After delivery the new born and the mother are immediately isolated from the rest of the household so that they do not come into contact with the other family members until after their first ritual bath. The first ritual bath takes place on the 9th day (this varies depending on the caste of the woman) after delivery. A separate bed is made with rags and mats for the mother and the new-born and the mother is given a separate set of utensils to use during this period of segregation and she has to wash and clean her own utensils after use because these things also become polluted and impure after the mother touches them.

This chapter presents and discusses the socio-cultural practices observed immediately after childbirth and delivery, during lactation, and the cultural reasons for abstinence both during pregnancy and immediately after delivery.

Practices After Delivery

In many traditional societies of the world, death, birth and other personal and family events entail danger and lead to the seclusion of affected persons, to prohibitions against contact and avoidance of certain foods or actions. In India persons affected in this way are impure for a period of time. Women are more impure than men, and childbirth and death cause temporary impurity to those close relatives whose natural substances are affected. In such cases purity can be restored by bathing, preferably, in the sacred water of the river Ganges, or at least in running water, tonsuring and abstaining from certain foodstuffs (Refer to chapter 2).

Though childbirth is a joyous occasion, nevertheless, it is regarded as impure and polluting, particularly for the mother and the new-born. Therefore, to prevent the entire household from being polluted and impure, normally the mother and the baby are isolated from the main house and from the ongoing activities for a certain period of time.

This polluting factor is very much in evidence in the study population, particularly after childbirth. In Motipur, 50 per cent immediately segregate

151

the mother and the new-born to either a separate room, if available, or to a corner of the living room, kitchen or the verandah, where the mother and the baby would not be in direct contact with other persons in the household. About a third of the respondents wash or bathe/sponge the mother and the child with hot water before segregation. Likewise in Kapgari, Santoshpur and Sultanpur, a majority immediately segregate the mother and the new-born to avoid the polluting effects of childbirth. See table 7.1.

Table 7.1:   Practices immediately after childbirth

PRACTICES AFTER CHILDBIRTH	MOTIPUR (Tribal)	KAPGARI (Hindu)	SANTOSHPUR (Muslim)	SULTANPUR (Developed)	TOTAL
IMMEDIATE SEGREGATION	49 (50%)	45 (45.91%)	89 (96.73%)	91 (96.80%)	274 (71.72%)
WASH/BATHE THEN SEPARATE	30 (30.61%)	31 (31.63%)	1 (1.08%)	1 (1.06%)	63 (16.49%)
OBSERVE RITUALS	1 (1.02%)	1 (1.02%)	-	1 (1.06%)	3 (0.78%)
OTHER	18 (18.36%)	21 (21.42%)	2 (2.17%)	1 (1.06%)	42 (10.99%)
TOTAL	98	98	92	94	382

Almost 97 per cent of the women in Sultanpur were immediately separated after childbirth from the rest of the household. This is because almost two thirds of the deliveries in this village were institutionalised and when women return home from the health centres after delivery, they are immediately segregated because of the polluting factor. But in Santoshpur, where nearly 70 per cent of the births were conducted at home, the women are kept in the same delivery room for the entire period of their seclusion. This high level of immediate segregation in both the villages of Sultanpur and Santoshpur can be because of their staunch and rigid belief in impurity/pollution after childbirth.

The period of seclusion depends on a number of factors. The most important is that of caste and religion. However, nowadays it also depends on the economic value and economic contribution of the mother towards the household income. As Mines (1989) observed, persons who become temporarily impure due to menstruation or a birth and death in the family are unable to perform certain duties. But, based on the person's status in the caste hierarchy or the person's occupational class, place of residence and socio-economic status in the community, the time length of incapacity varied. The Hindu higher caste women strictly observe seclusion for about three weeks, whilst women belonging to the lower caste observe it for about nine days, and the Muslims follow it for forty days. Depending on caste, religion, socio-economic and socio-cultural backgrounds and social standing of the household in the community, the period of isolation varies. As women's health care behaviour is partly related to pollution taboos, which is embedded in the wider socio-cultural context of the society, they are more or less governed by these concepts, as pollution is considered to be a powerful phenomena. Ullrich (1992), in a study of the Havik Brahmins in a southern Indian village found that taboos to have decreased in importance as a woman's primary role has been redefined as a marital partner rather than as a bearer of children. When her function was as a bearer of children, she was considered subject to biological rhythms and a threat to male ritual status. But with increased education, professional opportunities, and increased age at marriage for women, ritual status and male dominance have become less significant. Women are ritually less dangerous and less dependent on men, and transcend the biological rhythm that menstrual taboos symbolise.

The study found that a majority (83%) of the women in Motipur had a very small length of segregation period. This is almost certainly because most of the tribal women work outside home, as daily wage labourers, or along with their husbands in the fields, and if these women took a long time off from economic activity, their household income would be affected and hence they had a small period of confinement.

However, the other study villages reveal a somewhat different pattern. In Kapgari, 54 per cent of the women remained in seclusion between 21 to 31 days. Whereas, in Santoshpur, a majority (89%), remained in segregation for about 21 to 45 days because of their religious doctrine. But in Sultanpur, 41 per cent remained in isolation for about a fortnight, and 58 per cent observed it for a month. This is because most of the households in Sultanpur are nuclear and the women are indispensable as they are required to do most of the household chores, attend to the family's needs, care for children, cook, wash, etc.

The study found the resting period of women in Motipur to be rather small as compared to the other villages, where despite being in a joint family system, a woman's economic importance outweighs all other criteria related to her health and well being for the family to allow her to remain in seclusion for too long.

Reasons for Segregation

The main reason for isolating the mother and the child from the rest of the family immediately after childbirth is because of the "impurity and polluting effects of childbirth", according to 47 per cent of the surveyed women. The following accounts documented from case studies strongly illustrate the extent of belief in the concept of impurity and pollution after child birth.

> Someone was sent to fetch the *dai* during my labour pains, but in the meantime, I had given birth. No one attended to me, or attempted to clean me or my baby. I was lying on the mud floor in a pool of blood and placenta with the baby still attached to the umbilical cord. Eventually the *dai* arrived after an hour, cut the cord and cleaned me and my baby.
>
> Since my last child was delivered at home by relatives, they did not think it was necessary to call the *dai* so late at night, since I delivered my baby at 2 a.m. The *dai* was sent for in the morning to cut the cord and to clean me and my baby.

For details refer to table 7.2 which presents the reasons for segregation of the mother and the new-born baby.

Table 7.2:   Reasons for segregation

REASONS FOR SEGREGATION	MOTIPUR (Tribal)	KAPGARI (Hindu)	SANTOSHPUR (Muslim)	SULTANPUR (Developed)	TOTAL
MOTHER'S POLLUTING & IMPURE	80	85	7	8	180 (47.12%)
TO RECUPERATE & BE AWAY FROM INFECTIONS	18	13	38	55	124 (32.46%)
TRADITION/CUSTOM	-	-	2	31	33 (8.63%)
BLEEDING AFTER DELIVERY IS POLLUTING	-	-	45	-	45 (11.78%)
TOTAL	98	98	92	94	382

The table shows that more than four-fifths of the women in Motipur and Kapgari believe in the polluting factor. Whereas the women in Santoshpur considered the blood to be polluting, therefore they were secluded after childbirth because of bleeding. Whilst in Sultanpur, about a third of the respondents observed segregation as a custom and tradition.

In all the villages, a strong belief in pollution and impurity after child birth exists. But the length of segregation, type of place and kind of facilities and amenities given to the mother and the baby varies considerably from one place to another and also between different communities and caste groups. The general trend is to:

> Make a bed in a far corner of any available space (preferably far removed from the main house), on the mud floor with straw and hay, on top of which a mat is placed for the mother, and for the infant some rags are added on the mat. The mother is not given a pillow, or a blanket, or a bed sheet and has to sleep on this makeshift bed during her seclusion period, or until her first ritual bath. The

mother is also given a separate set of utensils to use during this period, which is thrown away after the completion of the segregation period. Almost all the things used by the mother during her confinement are discarded afterwards because of the polluting effects.

As pollution can be dangerous, enormous effort is made to avoid it spreading to the other family members, and utmost care is taken to choose such a place in the house so that the mother is not in direct contact with anybody during her confinement, and is as far removed from the main house as possible. Generally, the practice is to keep both the mother and the baby in a separate room (if available) and no one visits them except an elderly female relative of the household. In circumstances where spare rooms are unavailable, the mother and the baby are kept in a far corner of the living room, or the kitchen, or the verandah. The choice of place is largely dependent on the size of the house, number of rooms and number of family members. Table 7.3 presents the data on kind of place chosen for seclusion.

Table 7.3: **Kind of place chosen for segregation**

VILLAGE	SEPARATE ROOM	ROOM CORNER	KITCHEN CORNER	VERANDAH	TOTAL
MOTIPUR (Tribal, N_1 = 98)	41 (41.83%)	21 (21.42%)	21 (21.42%)	15 (15.30%)	98
KAPGARI (Hindu, N_2 = 98)	74 (75.51%)	10 (10.20%)	8 (8.16%)	6 (6.12%)	98
SANTOSHPUR (Muslim, N_3 = 92)	77 (83.69%)	10 (10.86%)	-	5 (5.43%)	92
SULTANPUR (Developed, N_4 = 94)	88 (93.61%)	4 (4.25%)	2 (2.12%)	-	94
TOTAL (N_T = 382)	280 (73.29%)	45 (11.78%)	31 (8.11%)	26 (6.80%)	382

As mentioned earlier persons affected by either birth or death in India avoid contact with persons and avoids certain foodstuffs considered to be harmful during this period. Hence, there are strict food taboos for women immediately after delivery and most of the women in the study population strictly adhered to it irrespective of religion, caste, and geographical location.

Food Avoidance

The daily diet of rural women is seldom nutritionally adequate; it becomes less so during pregnancy and lactation and after childbirth due to cultural taboos and restrictions regarding food intake and food avoidance. The same has been found in the study villages also.

> After delivery for the first three days I was on a diet of dry food, such as rice crisps, garlic, and *ghee* (clarified butter), and was allowed to eat only once, as this diet helps to contract the uterus quickly.

The study found that in both Motipur and Kapgari, immediately after delivery for the first three days the mothers are not given anything substantial to eat, except rice crisps with tea and hot water. On the fourth day when the woman has her ritual bath and clips her nails (she is assumed to be purified through this process), she is given rice and boiled vegetables, lentils and so on (depending on the economic status of the household), once a day. From this day onwards the mother eats one meal a day till the last day of her seclusion period.

The study found that the mothers are not given a proper meal for the first three days immediately after delivery. However, this practice varies from village to village depending on the caste and religion. The upper caste Hindu women have a longer period of restricted diet as opposed to the women from the lower castes. Muslim women too have a longer period of restricted diet after childbirth.

> For the first three days following delivery, I was only given rice crisps, a type of lentil, garlic, and *ghee* to eat. This kind of diet helps to recover quickly from childbirth. The elders of the household and the *dai* said that the amount of blood I lost during delivery and after delivery will be revived soon if I follow the diet pattern rigidly. Moreover, this kind of diet also helps in contracting the womb right away. I was allowed one proper mid-day meal on the 4th day after delivery, which consisted of boiled vegetables, lentils and rice. After the 4th day meal I was not given anything substantial to eat until the 9th day. On the 9th day after my first ritual bath I was allowed to eat a mid-day meal of rice and some boiled vegetables. Then again on the 13th day I was allowed to bathe again and clip my nails for purification. That day I was given a mid-day meal. Usually in evenings I was given rice crisps and tea. Until the 21st day I was kept on a diet of rice crisps, tea and hot water. After the 21st day, after my bath and the other rituals, I was allowed to eat two proper meals.

According to the women in Motipur, prohibitions and avoidance of foodstuffs nowadays depend mostly on the women's socio-cultural and socio-economic status. Around 30 per cent of the women in Motipur had one meal a day consisting of rice and different types of boiled vegetables and lentils, and in the night had rice crisps, tea and hot water. It is said this kind of diet helps contract the uterus quickly. About 40 per cent of the women were on a diet of dry foodstuff. Food which contains starch and water, like rice, potatoes, bananas, etc., are considered to be cold food and if taken immediately after childbirth, the mother develops a cold and passes it to the new-born through the breast milk. Very few women in this village ate a normal diet immediately after delivery.

In Kapgari also the women avoided certain food immediately after delivery. More than half of the women were on a diet of dry foodstuff which is presumed to help heal the body quickly and bring back the uterus to a normal position much faster. Around 16 per cent of the women had one meal a day, the mid-day meal, consisting of rice, boiled vegetables, or lentils/pulses, and in the evenings had rice crisps, tea and hot water. The women believed that if two meals are taken immediately after childbirth, both the mother and the child would be ill, and as rice is considered to be cold it is avoided at night. Only about 17 per cent of the surveyed women ate normally and did not observe the taboo of eating once a day.

In Santoshpur the mothers are allowed to eat only those foodstuff considered to be good for her and her child's health. Nearly three quarters of the surveyed women ate rice and boiled vegetables once a day. In the evenings they had rice crisps, tea, and hot water. This kind of diet continues till the last day of the segregation period, which is up to 40 days in the Muslim community. In Sultanpur 78 per cent of the women ate everything once a day for the entire period of seclusion, and 17 per cent had rice crisps, tea and hot water for the specified length of segregation.

The belief patterns in the study area are quite similar and the women believe that if the mother eats two meals a day consisting of foodstuff considered to be cold, both the mother and baby would be ill, the mother would not lactate properly and mother's body will take a longer time to recover and the uterus may not be normal again and the bleeding will continue for a long period of time. Because of these beliefs restricted diet is given to the mothers immediately after childbirth. This kind of diet continues till the woman is in seclusion. Only after that period is up, is she allowed to eat two times daily, but again, depending on the health of the child, the diet is changed constantly. Refer to table 7.4 for more details on reasons for restricted and prohibitive diet after delivery.

Table 7.4:   Reasons for restricted diet after delivery

REASONS FOR RESTRICTED DIET AFTER DELIVERY	MOTIPUR (Tribal)	KAPGARI (Hindu)	SANTOSHPUR (Muslim)	SULTANPUR (Developed)	TOTAL
TO RECOVER FROMCHILDBIRTH	25 (25.51%)	31 (31.63%)	9 (9.78%)	24 (25.53%)	89 (23.29%)
TRADITION/CUSTOM	13 (13.26%)	20 (20.40%)	8 (8.69%)	2 (2.12%)	43 (11.25%)
IT IS HARMFUL FOR/TO THE BABY	15 (15.30%)	19 (19.38%)	3 (3.26%)	2 (2.12%)	39 (10.20%)
TO IMPROVE MOTHER'S HEALTH	31 (31.63%)	22 (22.44%)	11 (11.95%)	63 (67.02%)	127 (33.24%)
TO INCREASE THE QUANTITY OF BREAST MILK	14 (14.28%)	-	-	2 (2.12%)	16 (4.18%)
DOCTOR'S ADVICE	-	1 (1.02%)	-	1 (1.06%)	2 (0.52%)
MOTHER & THE CHILD MIGHT CATCH COLD	-	-	39 (42.39%)	-	39 (10.20%)
DON'T KNOW	-	5 (5.10%)	22 (23.91%)	-	27 (7.06%)
TOTAL	98	98	92	94	382

During this period, generally the food items avoided are sugar, salt, vegetable oil, sour foods, fish, meat, eggs, pumpkins, eggplants, okra, drumsticks, etc. Some of the green leafy vegetables and various varieties of spinach are also forbidden to be taken immediately after delivery. Prawns and other sea-food are also prohibited as they apparently cause rheumatism and arthritis for the mother if taken immediately after childbirth. Mothers are given lots of garlic to enhance the process of "drying of the womb" (contraction of the uterus).

If a woman gives birth to a male child then she has to observe more taboos and restrictions with regards food intake. She is not allowed any green leafy vegetables, spinach, certain kinds of fish, pumpkin, spring onions, egg-plants, gourds, sour foods, fruits, etc. because of the belief that the infant will have loose bowels and acidity. Whereas if a woman gives birth to a female child she does not have to follow all the taboos and restrictions as rigorously because of the belief that a female infant is stronger and nothing can happen to her. The tradition of eating less and a different kind of diet for 21 days following delivery is in the best interest of the infant's and mother's health.

Hence, it can be concluded that a majority of the women believe in the theory of pollution and impurity after childbirth, and others believe that segregation is necessary to recuperate and to be away from infections. Therefore they remain in seclusion for a specified length of time. In addition they avoid certain foodstuffs known to be harmful for their health and their infants. Furthermore, they are on a restricted diet during that time period. Menstruation is also known to be polluting in the study villages.

Abstinence During Pregnancy and After Delivery

A belief persists in the rural areas that abstinence during pregnancy should be observed in order to have a safe delivery and a healthy baby. People believe that during pregnancy any conjugal relationship could jeopardise the child in the womb and both the mother and the baby could be hurt severely if abstinence is not observed, especially during the last few months. Hence, abstinence is practised quite rigidly. Some observe abstinence during the entire term of pregnancy, others follow either during the first or the last trimester of pregnancy, depending on the belief pattern existing in the area. Moreover, abstinence is also observed after childbirth for a certain period of time to safeguard both the mother and the child from any harmful side effects. The practice of sending pregnant women to their natal homes for delivery is also followed in most parts of the country, both in the rural and the urban areas. Women remain in their natal homes even after delivery. This is an indirect way of enforcing abstinence both during pregnancy and also after delivery.

Most women in the study villages practised abstinence both during pregnancy and after delivery. The practice of sending pregnant women to their natal homes for deliveries varied a great deal between villages, especially between the first and subsequent births. Refer to Table No. 7.5 for more details.

Table 7.5: **Practice of sending pregnant women to natal homes**

VILLAGE	FOR FIRST BIRTH	FOR EACH BIRTH	PRACTICE NOT FOLLOWED	TOTAL
MOTIPUR (Tribal)	1 (1.02%)	-	97 (98.97%)	98
KAPGARI (Hindu)	4 (4.08%)	8 (8.16%)	86 (87.75%)	98
SANTOSHPUR (Muslim)	54 (58.69%)	21 (22.82%)	17 (18.47%)	92
SULTANPUR (Developed)	24 (25.53%)	26 (27.65%)	44 (46.80%)	94
TOTAL	83 (21.72%)	55 (14.39%)	244 (63.87%)	382

The table indicates that in 22 per cent of the cases the practice of sending pregnant women to their natal homes for the first birth is followed. More than half follow this practice in Santoshpur, followed by a quarter in Sultanpur. This practice normally depends on the socio-economic condition of the woman's family and the custom and tradition of that particular community and caste group. In most instances this is normally followed only for the first birth and it is a custom and tradition in most of the communities in India. A majority of the women said the practice was good because they were more at ease at their natal place, had more rest, care, love and support from their own family and did not feel inhibited.

Abstinence is practised widely during pregnancy irrespective of religious beliefs, caste, tribe and geographical location. The study found that three quarters of the women observed abstinence during pregnancy. See table 7.6 for more information on abstinence during pregnancy.

Table 7.6:   Abstinence during pregnancy

VILLAGE	ABSTINENCE PRACTICED DURING PREGNANCY (%)		TOTAL
	YES	NO	
MOTIPUR (Tribal)	78	24	102
KAPGARI (Hindu)	79	21	100
SANTOSHPUR (Muslim)	69	31	100
SULTANPUR (Developed)	76	24	100
TOTAL	302 (75.12%)	100 (24.87%)	402

In villages Kapgari, Motipur and Sultanpur, women strictly followed abstinence during pregnancy. The women who follow abstinence are either more faithful in their belief or live in a joint family system, where the mother in law or any other elderly female relative monitors and controls the movement of pregnant daughter-in-law.

The data reveals that about 45 per cent and 43 per cent of the surveyed women from the villages of Motipur and Kapgari abstain from any conjugal relations both during the first and the second trimester of pregnancy. Whereas, in the other two villages of Santoshpur (42%) and Sultanpur (67%) women practice abstinence from either the sixth or seventh month of pregnancy, that is the last trimester. See table 7.7 for more information.

Table 7.7:   Period of abstinence during pregnancy

VILLAGE	HOW LONG IS ABSTINENCE PRACTICED DURING PREGNANCY					
	ENTIRE TERM	1ST TRIMESTER	1ST & 2ND TRIMESTER	NOT FOLLOWED AT ALL	OTHERS	TOTAL
MOTIPUR (Tribal)	-	15	45	24	18	102
KAPGARI (Hindu)	3	15	43	21	18	100
SANTOSHPUR (Muslim)	-	4	23	31	42	100
SULTANPUR (Developed)	6	3	-	24	67	100
TOTAL	9 (2.23%)	37 (9.20%)	111 (27.61%)	100 (24.87%)	145 (36.06%)	402

The differences in practising abstinence during pregnancy are because of different belief patterns existing in different communities. The women in Motipur and Kapgari believe that maintaining conjugal relations during the earlier stages of pregnancy leads to miscarriages or spontaneous abortions. The women in Santoshpur and Sultanpur believe that conjugal relations at a later stage of pregnancy harms both the mother and the child. According to them abstinence should be practised during the last few months of the pregnancy, because the baby is well developed and is a complete human being. At this stage to continue with conjugal relations will hurt the baby irreparably, and as a result it will be born deformed or with some defects.

However, besides fear, quite a large number of women maintained that it was not possible to continue with normal relations during the last trimester of pregnancy, as the mother grows too big and it becomes cumbersome and difficult to maintain normal relations. The reasons given for practising abstinence during pregnancy were varied and many. See table 7.8 for more details.

Table 7.8: **Reasons for abstinence during pregnancy**

REASONS FOR ABSTINENCE DURING PREGNANCY	MOTIPUR (Tribal)	KAPGARI (Hindu)	SANTOSHPUR (Muslim)	SULTANPUR (Developed)	TOTAL
MOTHER FEELS UNCOMFORTABLE & UNEASY	62	49	28	11	150 (37.31%)
DUE TO DIZZINESS, WEAKNESS & VOMITING	4	9	-	-	13 (3.23%)
MOTHER & THE CHILD COULD BE SEVERELY HURT	12	19	39	65	135 (33.58%)
DOCTOR'S ADVICE	-	2	2	-	4 (0.99%)
NOT PRACTICED AT ALL	24	21	31	24	100 (24.87%)
TOTAL	102	100	100	100	402

Table 7.8 reveals that 62 per cent of the women in Motipur said they were uncomfortable and felt uneasy (physically and psychologically) to continue with conjugal relations during pregnancy. Whilst, 65 per cent in Sultanpur were of the opinion that any normal relations could severely hurt the baby and the mother. Furthermore, 49 per cent of the women in Kapgari practised abstinence due to discomfort and uneasiness, and 39 per cent in Santoshpur also felt that continuing with normal relations could jeopardise the health of the mother and the baby, when the foetus is completely developed.

As mentioned earlier, abstinence is followed even after delivery for a number of reasons and the time length/period of abstinence after childbirth varies from individual to individual, depending on their belief, norms, values and also religion. It also depends on the fact whether the woman delivers at her natal home or at her husband's home. Refer to table 7.9 for more details.

Table 7.9: **How long abstinence practised after delivery**

HOW LONG ABSTINENCE PRACTICED AFTER DELIVERY	MOTIPUR (Tribal)	KAPGARI (Hindu)	SANTOSHPUR (Muslim)	SULTANPUR (Developed)	TOTAL
40-60 DAYS	31 (31.63%)	30 (30.61%)	42 (45.65%)	18 (19.14%)	121 (31.67%)
61-90 DAYS	22 (22.44%)	13 (13.26%)	-	36 (38.29%)	71 (18.58%)
91-120 DAYS	13 (13.26%)	26 (26.53%)	2 (2.17%)	14 (14.89%)	55 (14.39%)
121+ DAYS	29 (29.59%)	26 (26.53%)	43 (46.73%)	14 (14.89%)	112 (29.31%)
NOT PRACTICED AT ALL	2 (2.04%)	1 (1.02%)	5 (5.43%)	2 (2.12%)	10 (2.61%)
OTHERS	1 (1.02%)	2 (2.04%)	-	10 (10.63%)	13 (3.40%)
TOTAL	98	98	92	94	382

Very few women did not practice abstinence after delivery. Though a majority of the women observed abstinence, variations in the periods of abstinence were observed. Nonetheless, it was practised for at least 40-90 days in most cases. In Motipur and Kapgari, a majority of the women observed abstinence for about 40-60 days. Whereas in Santoshpur 47 per cent of the women observed abstinence after delivery for 121 days or more, and 38 per cent in Sultanpur practised abstinence after delivery for about 61-90 days.

The time length of this practice varies within the villages, but, nonetheless, it is practised and cuts across all barriers such as religion, caste, tribe, and so on. The reasons given for abstinence after delivery are varied but a majority of the women reckon it is because of the health of the mother, as she is weak immediately after childbirth and needs to recuperate before continuing with normal conjugal relations.

Though a large number of women observe and practice abstinence both during pregnancy and after childbirth, they seldom follow this practice during lactation. Only 11 per cent of the women in Kapgari and 2 per cent in Sultanpur observed abstinence during lactation. The women in Motipur and Santoshpur did not practice abstinence during lactation. Some women in Kapgari practised abstinence during lactation because of weakness, and a few thought it was harmful for the baby if the mother had a physical relationship. In Sultanpur it was practised because of fear of immediate pregnancy and because of weakness during lactation.

Cultural Practices Associated with Lactation

Food avoidance at the time of lactation is primarily perceived to be in the best interest of the baby, to whom harmful influences could be transmitted through the breast milk. Dietary restrictions deprive post-partum and lactating women of the nutritious ingredients at a time when they are particularly needed. The quality and quantity of breast milk is also adversely affected by such a diet.

Considering such belief patterns, most of the women in the study avoided certain kinds of food, which according to them were harmful for the infant. The foodstuffs avoided during the initial stages of lactation vary with age, religion, caste, economic status, and also varies from place to place producing distinct dietary patterns. The women in the study villages normally avoided food which according to them has laxative properties, food considered to be cold, food that causes skin rash or excema, and food which are acidic. Different social groups and communities have different norms which they follow during lactation.

A majority of the women had a normal diet during the initial stages of lactation, but a large number of them avoided altogether food items considered to be harmful for the baby. The food stuff avoided were certain green leafy vegetables, fibrous vegetables considered to have laxative properties, other vegetables like melon, gourds, egg plant, pumpkins, papayas, marrow's, which are considered to be 'hot', and food considered to be 'cold' such as rice, bananas, yoghurt. Other foods which are avoided during this period include any sour foods like oranges, grapes, lemon, lime and so on (these are considered to be acidic), and also oily and spicy food, chillies and peppers; any kind of shell fish, prawns, shrimps which cause indigestion. Many women also avoided eggs as they are considered to be very 'hot', which causes skin rash and boils. The women who avoided certain food during lactation said it was harmful for the infant's health. In Sultanpur women gave acidity as a reason for avoiding certain food items.

Very few women had any special food during the initial stages of lactation. Generally these women were from the upper socio-economic group, and the women who had delivered at their natal homes. More than three quarters of the women never consumed any special food during the initial stages of lactation. The women who had special food had items such as milk, eggs, fruits, various types of pulses and lentils, meat, fish, etc. The women in Sultanpur were also given an additional supplementary diet from their Anganwadi Centre. A majority of the women consumed special food to increase the quantity of breast milk and the others had special food to improve mother's health.

The food taboos and avoidance imposed on women during any period of their life are supposedly in the best interest of both the women and their infants, and to protect them from any impairment or ill health. In reality the taboos, prejudices, beliefs and attitudes centring around food are cultural practices that act as blocks preventing full utilisation of the available food which grows practically in every household kitchen garden of the study villages.

In the study villages certain cultural practices are still followed immediately after childbirth and during the initial stages of lactation which are harmful both for the mother and the new-born. Even though the women justify the cultural practices of segregation, restricted food intake and food avoidance after childbirth, these practices have detrimental impact on women's health. Close spaced pregnancies lead to a deterioration in women's health because of anaemia and malnutrition and due to belief patterns and cultural practices associated with pregnancy, childbirth, labour and delivery. Most of the home deliveries take place in unhygienic conditions and immediate segregation of the mothers to dim and squalid corners without any adequate diet can lead to various infections and can affect her health adversely. In addition, prolonged food avoidance and restricted diet is justified as a cultural practice depriving mothers of adequate nutrition and nourishment most needed after childbirth and during the initial stages of lactation. This causes irreparable damage both to the health of the mother and to the new-born child.

Conclusion

The study presents evidence that certain cultural practices followed after delivery and childbirth affect both the mothers and the child's health directly in a detrimental way. Programme and policy initiatives are necessary to enhance the quality of maternal health to reduce mortality and morbidity of mothers. Programmes should be developed to discourage segregation of mother to unhygienic places and corners after childbirth. Besides, institutionalised deliveries should be encouraged, and supplementary diet should be provided for the mothers through the PHCs and their Integrated Child Development Scheme (ICDS). Postnatal services should be provided at homes by the health centres in view of compulsory confinement of the mothers immediately after childbirth. Health education programmes should take these cultural practices into consideration.

Health Status of Children

Radha is 24 years old and has three children, two daughters and a son. Her son was born three months prior to the survey, and she says he was bigger than the average size. Since her last delivery was at the health centre, she remembers her son being weighed after birth. However, she can not remember the exact weight at birth but believes it was around 3000 grams. Immediately after the birth, her son was given hot water at the hospital after a few hours. She breast-fed him after four days as she had insufficient milk. Even though, she is still breast feeding her son, she says that she has very little milk, therefore she has started giving supplementary food to the infant from the first month itself (sago and fresh milk). She says she weaned her daughters after one year, but started giving supplementary food from the fourth month itself in the form of fresh milk, sago, mushy food, plain water, etc.

Even though she had insufficient milk for breast feeding, none the less, during lactation she avoided sour foods, certain kinds of green leafy vegetables, fibrous vegetables, and also other types of vegetables, certain kinds of fish, chillies, cold water and cold rice. She says if she does not avoid these food items, her child would catch cold and get fever and have very loose bowels. However, despite following these practices rigidly, her son is not keeping well and is intermittently plagued with fever, cough and cold, and sometimes has bouts of severe vomiting. She is very worried and has also reduced her food intake fearing that this is what is making her child ill, as they are allowed to eat little quantity of food in the best interest of the child's and mother's health.

It is a well documented fact that mother's abilities and health are important for the child's health, and survival (Refer to Chapter 2 for more information). This chapter is divided into three main sections. Section I presents the reproductive status of the surveyed women and mortality of infants and children. Section II describes the health status of infants and children and outlines the information on birth weight, breast feeding and weaning practices. Section III describes the health care utilisation pattern and behaviour, especially immunisation for infants and children, and health care utilisation during minor and common ailments of childhood and infancy.

SECTION I

This section primarily details the reproductive status of the mothers, and children ever born to them. It also gives information on stillbirths, abortions, both spontaneous and induced, sex preference, birth status of the children, sex ratio, and infant and childhood mortality.

Reproduction and Children Ever Born

In the developing countries of the world, since women marry at an earlier age, especially in the rural areas, their reproductive cycle begins relatively earlier than most educated urban women. In most of the rural areas of India women marry after attaining puberty, but in some parts of the country, particularly in rural north India, sometimes they marry even before the attainment of menarche.

After marriage the woman moves in with her husband and his family. To prove her right of abode at her in-laws she has to give birth to a son to carry on the family lineage, and thus begins her entry into a vicious cycle of reproduction immediately after marriage to produce a male child. A woman faces untold risks to have a male child, and keeps having children against all odds to produce a son.

This trend was observed in the study villages also. The most desired family size of most women was that of two living sons and a daughter. The women with lower levels of educational attainment or no schooling married earlier than women with a few years of schooling. Very few women married in their early or mid twenties. Nearly 48 per cent of the total women were married between the ages of 15-19 years, and 32 per cent between the ages of 8-14 years (See Chapter 4). As a majority of the women start having children when they are very young, most of them complete their desired family size by 25-30 years of age. However, those women who cannot achieve their desired family keep bearing children even at an advanced age to have a son to carry the family lineage. Due to repeated childbearing and close-spaced pregnancies, many women had stillborn babies, miscarriages and spontaneous abortions. Very few women voluntarily had a pregnancy terminated. See table 8.1.

Table 8.1: **Percentage stillbirths**

VILLAGE	EVER HAD A STILLBIRTH	No. OF STILLBIRTHS			TOTAL
		ONE	TWO	FOUR	
MOTIPUR (Tribal, N_1 = 98)	9 (9.18%)	4	4	1	9
KAPGARI (Hindu, N_2 = 98)	9 (9.18%)	8	1	-	9
SANTOSHPUR (Muslim, N_3=92)	12 (13.04%)	8	4	-	12
SULTANPUR (Developed, N_4= 94)	4 (4.25%)	4	-	-	4
TOTAL (N_T = 382)	34 (8.90%)	24 (70.58%)	9 (26.47%)	1 (2.94%)	34

Around nine per cent of the total women had stillborn babies. The table indicates that women in Santoshpur had maximum number of stillbirths. This is because age of mother has a significant association with stillbirths and children ever born. Miscarriages, abortions and stillbirths are more frequent among younger and older women. Furthermore, women bear children at regular intervals and the spacing between children is very small. In general, poor health of the mother, anaemia during pregnancy, nutritional status, workload, etc. also affect the viability of a baby. The lowest number of stillbirths recorded was for women in Sultanpur.

Table 8.2: **Percentage abortions**

VILLAGE	EVER HAD AN ABORTION	SPONTANEOUS ABORTION			INDUCED ABORTIONS	
		ONE	TWO	THREE	ONE	TWO
MOTIPUR (Tribal, N_{11} =102)	6	2	2	1	1	-
KAPGARI (Hindu, N_{22} =100)	5	3	-	-	2	-
SANTOSHPUR (Muslim, N_{33} =100)	19	13	5	-	-	1
SULTANPUR (Developed, N_4 =100)	22	6	7	-	6	3
TOTAL (N_{TT}= 402)	52 (12.93%)	24 (46.15%)	14 (26.92%)	1 (1.92%)	9 (17.30%)	4 (7.69%)

Overall 13 per cent of the women had an abortion. The maximum number of abortions (both spontaneous and induced) was reported in Sultanpur. The women in Santoshpur had the highest number of spontaneous abortions followed by Sultanpur. Few women in Kapgari and Motipur had spontaneous abortions.

Table 8.3: **Percentage sex preference**

VILLAGE	CURRENTLY PREGNANT	SEX PREFERENCE			SEX PREFERENCE DURING LAST PREGNANCY	
		MALE	FEMALE	D.K	MALE	FEMALE
MOTIPUR (Tribal, N_1 =102)	20	11 (55%)	6 (30%)	3 (15%)	78	24
KAPGARI (Hindu, N_2 =100)	12	7 (58%)	3 (25%)	2 (17%)	72	28
SANTOSHPUR (Muslim, N_3 =100)	20	9 (45%)	5 (25%)	6 (30%)	85	14
SULTANPUR (Developed, N_4 =100)	6	2 (33%)	2 (33%)	2 (33%)	74	26
TOTAL (N_T = 402)	58 (14.42%)	29 (50%)	18 (31.03%)	13 (22.41%)	309 (76.86%)	92(22.88%)

The table shows that 14 per cent of the total women were pregnant at the time of the survey. One half of the total women who were currently pregnant wanted a male child as opposed to 31 per cent who wanted a female child, whereas 22 per cent of the currently pregnant women were not sure about their preference. However, a majority of the women from all villages wanted a male child as opposed to a third of the women in Sultanpur. Moreover, a large percentage (77%) of the total women wanted a male child during their last pregnancy as opposed to 23 per cent who wanted a female child.

More single births were reported, multiple births were very few. The women in Santoshpur had the maximum number of multiple births followed by Kapgari and Motipur respectively. No multiple births were reported in Sultanpur. See table 8.4 for more details.

Table 8.4:   Birth status

VILLAGE	SINGLE BIRTHS	MULTIPLE BIRTHS	TOTAL
MOTIPUR (Tribal)	290 (99.31%)	2 (0.68%)	292
KAPGARI (Hindu)	291 (97.97%)	6 (2.02%)	297
SANTOSHPUR (Muslim)	300 (97.40%)	8 (2.59%)	308
SULTANPUR (Developed)	221 (100%)	-	221
TOTAL	1102 (98.56%)	16 (1.43%)	1118

More male children were recorded at birth in all the villages. The difference between male and female children at birth was quite high in most villages with the sole exception of village Sultanpur which revealed only one more male child than the females. See table 8.5.

Table 8.5:   Sex of the child at birth

VILLAGE	SEX OF THE CHILD		TOTAL
	MALE	FEMALE	
MOTIPUR (Tribal, N_1 =102)	162 (55.47%)	130 (44.52%)	292
KAPGARI (Hindu, N_2 =100)	175 (58.92%)	122 (41.07%)	297
SANTOSHPUR (Muslim, N_3 =100)	199 (64.61%)	109 (35.38%)	308
SULTANPUR (Developed, N_4=100)	111 (50.22%)	110 (49.77%)	221
TOTAL (N_T = 402)	647 (57.87%)	471 (42.12%)	1118

Sex ratio at birth is always slightly higher for male babies. There is no 1:1 conformity in the male and female births. It is generally 105 male babies per 100 female babies. According to the Health Information India-1990, the Sex Ratio for West Bengal is:

Total- 911 females per 1000 males

Rural- 947 females per 1000 males

Urban- 819 females per 1000 males

"Unlike most other regions of the world, males outnumber females. This is especially striking among the 200 million or so people of the north-western states of Punjab, Haryana, Rajasthan and Uttar Pradesh" (Jeffery, Jeffery and Lyon, 1989).

According to a study done by Jeffery et. al. in two rural districts and villages of Uttar Pradesh, they found that women's experiences in Bijnor District basically reflected this pattern of more males. They further found that in rural Uttar Pradesh as a whole female death rates at all ages up to 40 exceeded male death rates. Excess female mortality, in combination with excess male births, results in a skewed sex ratio. The 1981 Census recorded 886 females for every 1000 males in Uttar Pradesh. The Bijnor District figures showed an even greater disparity, with just 863 females for every 1000 males (Jeffery, Jeffery, and Lyon, 1989).

The table shows that the birth of more male children was recorded in all the study villages, but more so in the villages of Santoshpur, Kapgari and Motipur respectively. Reportedly there were 90 more male children at birth in Santoshpur as opposed to one in Sultanpur. Similarly, there were 53 more male children at birth in Kapgari, and 32 more male children in Motipur.

Gender inequality is an important indicator of discrimination against females and is an indicator of son-preference in societies. Although skewed sex ratio has been observed in the study villages, due to lack of adequate and appropriate data to explain this phenomena, the following postulations are put forth which might help explain this skewed sex ration to a certain extent.

Sex Selective Abortions (Amniocentesis)

This is a relatively new technology in the rural parts of India and is accessible mostly in the urban areas. It is also a relatively expensive technology by rural standards.

Infanticide

Infanticide is still a common practice in several states of India (especially in the Northern States), but there is no direct evidence of infanticide in the study villages and in West Bengal it is not very well documented. This practice is generally carried out by the *dais* at the instruction of the male members of the household or elderly (senior) female members at birth. Often times, this practice is done without the knowledge of the mother. Data on infanticide is hard to come by as people are not willing to talk about this practice. I tried to probe into this during the field work and I explored this further by interviewing several health workers from the PHCs and *dais* with a view to generate data to explain the skewed sex ratio. However, I do not have data to substantiate and can only hypothesise on the causes of skewed sex ratio.

Though no discrimination was observed in the study villages in seeking health care and medical attention for either a girl child or a male child, some gender based differences in health care utilisation was noticed. For girls allopathic treatment was sought, whereas for boys either homeopathic treatment or other traditional medicines were preferred because of the belief that boys are not strong enough to digest allopathic medicines. This "over-protection" of sons induces more male mortality in the study villages during childhood years as opposed to girl children.

Under Five Mortality

Though the sex ratio at birth is favourable towards male babies, death amongst the male babies within the first year of life is much higher than the female babies. The study reveals that out of the 70 babies who died, nearly 69 per cent were boys as opposed to 31 per cent of the female children. See table 8.6 for information.

Table 8.6:   **Number of deaths by sex of children**

VILLAGE	No. OF DEATHS BY SEX		TOTAL	TOTAL No. OF CHILDREN
	MALE	FEMALE		EVER BORN
MOTIPUR (Tribal)	6 (50%)	6 (50%)	12 (4.10%)	292
KAPGARI (Hindu)	9 (81.81%)	2 (18.18%)	11 (3.70%)	297
SANTOSHPUR (Muslim)	21 (80.76%)	5 (19.23%)	26 (8.44%)	308
SULTANPUR (Developed)	12 (57.14%)	9 (42.85%)	21 (9.50%)	221
TOTAL	48 (68.57%)	22 (31.42%)	70 (6.26%)	1118

According to the data more male babies died within the first year of their lives. A majority of the new-born babies died in their infancy (between day one to 364 days. See table 8.7 for more details.

Table 8.7: **Age at death of children by sex**

| VILLAGE | AGE AT DEATH OF THE CHILDREN BY SEX | | | | | | TOTAL No. OF DEATHS | TOTAL No. OF CEB |
| | 1 to 28 Days | | 1 Month to 12 Months | | From 1 Year to 5 Yrs. | | | |
	MALES	FEMALES	MALES	FEMALES	MALES	FEMALES		
MOTIPUR (Tribal)	1	3	1	3	4	-	12	292
KAPGARI (Hindu)	2	-	5	2	2	-	11	297
SANTOSHPUR (Muslim)	7	2	4	2	10	1	26	308
SULTANPUR (Developed)	1	2	3	4	8	3	21	221
TOTAL	11 (15.71%)	7 (10%)	13 (18.57%)	11 (15.71%)	24 (34.28%)	4 (5.71%)	70 (6.26%)	1118

Out of the total number (1118) of children ever born, six per cent died in their infancy and childhood years. Most of the deaths occurred in the childhood years (between one to five years of age) and in infancy. A quarter of the babies died within days after birth, that is, before completing the first month of their life (between 1 to 28 days).

The causes of infant deaths are generally due to maternal factors such as lack of antenatal and natal care; poor health of mother during pregnancy and lactation; age of mother, parity, spacing of births; nutritional status of mother during pregnancy; delivery problems and type of attendance and care at delivery; low birth weight babies; infant feeding practices; and so on. In addition, infant deaths can also be caused due to environmental and hygienic factors like unclean water and food; unsanitary disposal of wastage; water-borne disease (diarrhoea, dysentery, cholera, etc.), air-borne diseases like respiratory tract infection, fever; or social factors like the condition of the house, toilet facilities, crowding, quality of drinking water and source of fuel and lighting; social taboos; poverty and ignorance of the parents; lack of education of the mother; and economic conditions such as household income. The tests of association between various maternal factors like age of the mother, education, children ever born, antenatal care, place of delivery, income of the household, occupation, workload etc. do not show any significant relationship and association with the death of infants in the study population.

The overall fertility level was 2.78 children per woman. Most of the women had single births. The sex ratio at birth was favourable towards male babies, but more male babies died before completing the first year of their life. This is because male babies are not given immediate treatment during illness because of the myth that male babies are not strong enough to digest allopathic medicines, therefore they are treated with alternative and traditional medicines even during severe ailments. Hence male babies died more frequently in the study villages. Estimated infant mortality is approximately 62 per thousand live births.

SECTION II

Health Status of Infants and Children

This section of the study primarily focuses on health status and health care utilisation for children under the age of five years. All the information pertaining to this topic was gathered on the last child born to the women prior to the survey. In this section information on birth weight, breast feeding, weaning, supplementary diet, immunisation, illness is covered.

Since in general the women themselves are weak and undernourished because of repeated and close spaced pregnancies, the children born to them are normally of low birth weight and small for a full term baby. Several studies have highlighted the importance of age of the mother, parity, nutritional status, antenatal care during pregnancy, workload during pregnancy, and in general poor health of the mother affecting the birth weight of the babies. Several studies have also linked low weight at birth to mother's health and nutritional status at the time of pregnancy and also during her entire reproductive phase. Low birth weight reduces the chances of child survival, and an increase in perinatal mortality and short intervals between births is also detrimental to the health of both the mother and the child (Refer to chapter 2).

Therefore weight at birth of the last child was queried to see if age of the mother, parity, nutritional status, workload during pregnancy etc., had an effect on the birth weight of the children. The study found that many babies were not weighed at birth since a majority of the births were delivered at home by friends, relatives or *dais* (Refer to chapter 6). The study further shows that only four per cent of the infants were weighed at birth in Motipur, as compared to 66 per cent in Sultanpur. This is probably because a large number of births in Sultanpur were attended by trained health personnel at home as well as in the health centres and hospitals (Refer to chapter 6). Thirty per cent of the babies were weighed at birth in Kapgari followed by 18 per cent in Santoshpur. Refer to table 8.8 for details.

Table 8.8:   **New-born weighed at birth**

VILLAGE	WAS YOUR LAST CHILD WEIGHED AT BIRTH			TOTAL
	YES	NO	DON'T KNOW	
MOTIPUR (Tribal)	4 (4.08%)	90 (91.83%)	4 (4.08%)	98
KAPGARI (Hindu)	29 (29.59%)	57 (58.16%)	12 (12.24%)	98
SANTOSHPUR (Muslim)	17 (18.47%)	70 (76.08%)	5 (5.43%)	92
SULTANPUR (Developed)	62 (65.95%)	27 (28.72%)	5 (5.31%)	94
TOTAL	112 (29.31%)	244 (63.87%)	27 (7.06%)	382

Overall 29 per cent of the babies were weighed at birth. Even though a majority of the babies were not weighed at birth, the women, because of their experience in child bearing, guessed the size of their babies when they were born. About 43 per cent of the total women recalled that their babies were of average size at birth. Further, a quarter of the women said they had small babies and 28 per cent said they had large babies at birth. See table 8.9 for more details.

Table 8.9:   **Size of the new-born baby at birth**

| VILLAGE | WHAT WAS THE SIZE OF YOUR LAST CHILD AT BIRTH | | | | TOTAL |
	LARGE	AVERAGE	SMALL	DON'T KNOW	
MOTIPUR (Tribal)	17 (17.34%)	57 (58.16%)	19 (19.38%)	5 (5.10%)	98
KAPGARI (Hindu)	30 (30.61%)	48 (48.97%)	10 (10.20%)	10 (10.20%)	98
SANTOSHPUR (Muslim)	16 (17.39%)	33 (35.86%)	41 (44.56%)	2 (2.17%)	92
SULTANPUR (Developed)	43 (45.74%)	26 (27.65%)	23 (24.46%)	2 (2.17%)	94
TOTAL	106 (27.74%)	164 (42.93%)	93 (24.34%)	19 (4.97%)	382

A greater number of small babies were born to the mothers in Santoshpur, followed by Sultanpur. A large number of women from villages Motipur and Kapgari said they had average sized babies according to their impression (the standardised weight at birth according to the World Health Organisation is 2500 grams).

Those babies who were weighed at birth had a varied and wide distribution of birth weights; the smallest being 1500 grams and the largest being 5300 grams. Amongst all the surveyed babies weighed at birth, 30 per cent of the babies were of the recommended standardised birth weight of 2500 grams, 13 per cent were below the recommended birth weight and 56 per cent were more than 2500 grams (between 2750 grams to 5300 grams weight at birth).

The babies born to women in Sultanpur had a higher birth weight as compared to the other villages. The health, nutritional status, workload, of the mother, and the general socio-economic conditions of the household does affect the weight at birth. The study also found that household income, occupation of both husband and wife and religion are significantly associated and related with weight at birth. The test on mother's occupation and birth weight reveals a significant association [x^2=10.64; P≤0.05].

Where health of the new-born babies is concerned, breast feeding provides the best nutrition for the infants. The data shows that an overwhelming majority of the women breast-fed their babies for two years or more. Only a negligible minority (6%) did not or could not breast feed their infants. The reasons given for not breast feeding were that of 'Insufficient Milk' (36%), followed by 'Mother too weak/ill' to breast feed (23%) and the 'Child refused to Suckle' (32%) and so on.

Breast feeding is normally initiated after 24 to 72 hours in most parts of India. The same pattern has been observed in the study villages too. The infants were given some kind of pre-lacteal feeds before breast feeding. See table 8.10 for more information.

Table 8.10:   How long after birth put child to breast

VILLAGE	HOW LONG AFTER BIRTH FIRST STARTED BREAST FEEDING THE INFANT				TOTAL
	IMMEDIATELY	LESS THAN AN HOUR	LESS THAN 24 HOURS	OTHER	
MOTIPUR (Tribal)	-	1 (1.02%)	41 (41.83%)	56 (57.14%)	98
KAPGARI (Hindu)	4 (4.08%)	13 (13.26%)	26 (26.53%)	55 (56.12%)	98
SANTOSHPUR (Muslim)	-	21 (22.82%)	26 (28.26%)	45 (45.91%)	92
SULTANPUR (Developed)	15 (15.95%)	9 (9.57%)	43 (45.74%)	27 (28.72)	94
TOTAL	19 (4.97%)	44 (11.51%)	136 (35.60%)	183 (47.90%)	382

Quite a large proportion (48%) of women first started breast feeding three days after the birth, followed by more than a third who first put their child to the breast less than 24 hours after birth. The women who delayed breast feeding after childbirth gave a number of reasons for doing so, but the universal reason was that 'it was harmful for the baby' and that there was 'insufficient milk' to nurse the infants immediately after birth. More than a third of the women could not nurse because of insufficient milk and 28 per cent thought it was harmful for the baby. Furthermore, 17 per cent of the women were too weak after delivery to breast feed. Almost one half of the women squeezed colostrum before breast feeding.

Breast feeding was found to be universal and extended over a long period of time in the study population. A majority of the women nursed their babies for more than a year and even up to two to three years. The duration of breast feeding in most countries is longest among uneducated women who breast feed according to age-old traditions. Educated mothers, even if they attend school only for some years and did not even complete primary education, wean their child earlier. The present data also shows that with more years spent in school the frequency and length of breast feeding reduces [x^2=22.21; P≤0.05]. Due to modernisation and increase in the levels of education among women the duration of breast feeding is decreasing. Table 8.11 gives more detailed information on the time length of breast feeding.

Table 8.11: **How long breast-fed the last child**

HOW LONG BREASTFED YOUR LAST CHILD	MOTIPUR (Tribal)	KAPGARI (Hindu)	SANTOSHPUR (Muslim)	SULTANPUR (Developed)	TOTAL
LESS THAN A YEAR	-	-	18 (19.56%)	7 (7.44%)	25 (6.54%)
ONE YEAR	5 (5.10%)	7 (7.14%)	14 (15.21%)	18 (19.14%)	44 (11.51%)
TWO YEARS	12 (12.24%)	5 (5.10%)	-	-	17 (4.45%)
THREE YEARS	12 (12.24%)	6 (6.12%)	-	16 (17.02%)	34 (8.90%)
FOUR YEARS	16 (16.32%)	17 (17.34%)	-	6 (6.38%)	39 (10.20%)
FIVE YEARS	3 (3.06%)	2 (2.04%)	-	2 (2.12%)	7 (1.83%)
UNTIL CHILD DIED	2 (2.04%)	1 (1.02%)	-	3 (3.19%)	6 (1.57%)
NEVER BREAST FED	-	4 (4.08%)	1 (1.08%)	-	5 (1.30%)
STILL BREAST FEEDING	48 (48.97%)	56 (57.14%)	59 (64.13%)	42 (44.68%)	205 (53.66%)
TOTAL	98	98	92	94	382

A majority of the mothers nursed their babies between one to two years followed by three to four years. Many mothers stopped nursing their children because of insufficient milk or because the child refused to be breast fed. In addition, there were other reasons for not nursing, like the mother was too ill or weak, or the child was too ill or weak to suckle, or the child died during infancy. A negligible percentage of the mothers stopped breast feeding because they were gainfully employed.

Besides breast feeding, the infants and children are also given supplementary food at a certain age. For a female child supplementary food is introduced in the sixth month and for the male child in the seventh or the ninth month depending on various factors such as caste, religion, tribe and so on. Nevertheless, some kind of supplementary diet was given to all children. No gender discrimination was found in the study villages with regards breast feeding of infants, or in introducing supplementary food for the babies. See table 8.12 for reference on introduction of supplementary or additional food for babies.

Table 8.12: **Supplementary food given besides breast milk**

BESIDES BREAST MILK WAS THE CHILD GIVEN ANYTHING ELSE TO EAT OR DRINK	MOTIPUR (Tribal)	KAPGARI (Hindu)	SANTOSHPUR (Muslim)	SULTANPUR (Developed)	TOTAL
YES	89 (90.81%)	89 (90.81%)	79 (85.86%)	86 (91.48%)	343 (89.79%)
NO	9 (9.18%)	9 (9.18%)	12 (13.04%)	5 (5.31%)	35 (9.16%)
NOT APPLICABLE (CHILD DIED)	-	-	1 (1.08%)	3 (3.19%)	4 (1.04%)
TOTAL	98	98	92	94	382

An overwhelming 90 per cent of the women started some kind of supplementary food or drink for their children during infancy. In almost all the villages with the exception of Sultanpur, the babies were first introduced to additional food between the fourth and sixth month of their lives and were generally given plain water, fresh milk, baby formula or soft mushy food. The women in Sultanpur introduced supplementary food for the first time between the first and third month in the form of plain water, fresh milk, baby formula. Solid and soft mushy food were given between the age of four and six months. In addition, other liquids were also given to the infants like fruit and vegetable juice, clear soup, stew and so on.

Though breast feeding is universal in the study villages, it is not initiated until after 24 to 72 hours after birth, and during this time some pre-lacteal feed is given to the infants to cleanse its system of impurities. Time length of breast feeding varied according to the educational attainment and women with some years of schooling weaned their babies earlier than the uneducated mothers and decreased breast feeding considerably as opposed to illiterate mothers. The mothers with some schooling introduced supplementary food earlier than the mothers with no schooling. The overall birth weight of an infant was found to be dependent more on socio-economic condition of the household and various maternal factors. Most women had average or above sized babies.

SECTION III

Health Care Utilisation for Infants and Children

This part deals with the health care utilisation for infants and children (between the age of 0-5 years), particularly utilisation of immunisation services. Health care utilisation during minor and common ailments of childhood and infancy were also queried. The questions were mainly addressed to the mothers for the last living child born to the mothers prior to the survey.

All of Radha's children have been immunised against tuberculosis, polio, whooping cough and tetanus. The last child just got his BCG vaccination, and since he's been ill she could not take him to the polio clinic for the polio vaccine which is due and also for the other vaccinations.

She strongly believes in the supernatural, evil spirits, foul winds, etc. She often visits the village 'Ojha' for treatment. When her son was vomiting excessively she thought he was about to die and she took him to the 'Ojha' for treatment, instead of the hospital. She says her son was cured quite soon with the 'Ojha's' treatment. She says for certain ailments and illness, the 'Ojha's' treatment works, (for example, in case of excessive vomiting, excessive crying without any reason, and if a person is possessed by evil spirits, or is a victim of evil eyes and so on). However, for any other illness she always consults with a western doctor first (for daughters, she prefers allopathic medicine and for the son it is always homeopathic medicine). But if an illness is not cured within a short period of time, then she goes in for traditional treatment to the '*Ojha*'. She says she has used all the different medical facilities available simultaneously for her children and for herself.

When she and both her daughters were suffering from measles and chicken-pox they never consulted with any medical practitioners. During that time they practised certain rituals like eating only vegetarian food and keeping everything very clean (bed, house, yard, etc.). For seven days they are not supposed to eat food cooked in oil, or fish, garlic, onions, meat etc. at home. This is seen as a visitation by a goddess to their home. The patient is normally kept in a separate room (if available) and they light incense and pray to goddess '*Sitala*'. After seven days the patient is bathed with green (tender) coconut water. The popular belief is that pox and measles take a certain length of time to cure itself whether one consults a doctor or not, and therefore often patients are left alone to get well.

Villages Sultanpur and Kapgari were well covered by various immunisation services and programmes as opposed to the other two study villages. Motipur was very poorly covered by immunisation programmes and services. Refer to the table 8.13.

Table 8.13: **Child received any vaccination**

YOUR LAST CHILD EVER RECEIVED ANY OF THE FOLLOWING VACCINATIONS	MOTIPUR (Tribal)	KAPGARI (Hindu)	SANTOSHPUR (Muslim)	SULTANPUR (Developed)	TOTAL
RECEIVED BCG VACCINATION					
YES	28 (28.57%)	87 (88.77%)	60 (65.21%)	85 (90.42%)	260 (68.06%)
NO	60 (61.22%)	3 (3.06%)	22 (23.91%)	6 (6.38%)	91 (23.82%)
DON'T KNOW	10 (10.20%)	8 (8.16%)	10 (10.86%)	3 (3.19%)	31 (8.11%)
TOTAL	98	98	92	94	382
RECEIVED DPT VACCINATIONS					
YES	25 (25.51%)	74 (75.51%)	62 (67.39%)	85 (90.42%)	246 (64.39%)
NO	61 (62.24%)	12 (12.24%)	19 (20.65%)	6 (6.38%)	98 (25.65%)
DON'T KNOW	12 (12.24%)	12 (12.24%)	11 (11.95%)	3 (3.19%)	38 (9.94%)
TOTAL	98	98	92	94	382
RECEIVED POLIO VACCINE					
YES	33 (33.67%)	85 (86.73%)	62 (67.39%)	82 (87.23%)	262 (68.58%)
NO	48 (48.97%)	4 (4.08%)	19 (20.65%)	9 (9.57%)	80 (20.94%)
DON'T KNOW	17 (17.34%)	9 (9.18%)	11 (11.95%)	3 (3.19%)	40 (10.47%)
TOTAL	98	98	92	94	382
INJECTION AGAINST MEASLES					
YES	12 (12.24%)	38 (38.77%)	40 (43.47%)	65 (69.14%)	155 (40.57%)
NO	76 (77.55%)	32 (32.65%)	42 (45.65%)	22 (23.40%)	172 (45.02%)
DON'T KNOW	10 (10.20%)	28 (28.57%)	10 (10.86%)	7 (7.44%)	55 (14.39%)
TOTAL	98	98	92	94	382
RECEIVED DOSE OF VITAMIN A					
YES	3 (3.06%)	14 (14.28%)	40 (43.47%)	63 (67.02%)	120 (31.41%)
NO	85 (86.73%)	55 (56.12%)	43 (46.73%)	18 (19.14%)	201 (52.61%)
DON'T KNOW	10 (10.20%)	29 (29.59%)	9 (9.78%)	13 (13.82%)	61 (15.96%)
TOTAL WOMEN WITH CHILDREN	98	98	92	94	382

The table shows that 68 per cent of the total children below the age of five years were immunised against tuberculosis (BCG), and 64 per cent were immunised against diphtheria, whooping cough and tetanus (DPT). Though the overall immunisation coverage for both BCG and DPT vaccinations are more than 60 per cent, the villages if observed individually reveal an extensive variance in its immunisation coverage.

All the study villages have had access to health facilities within a radius of five kilometres, therefore, it seems that the people in Motipur did not utilise immunisation services for infants and children. This is because of ignorance or apathy towards immunisation programmes (though they are aware of the immunisation services available through the health centres).

Under utilisation of the polio vaccine was also found in Motipur as opposed to the other study villages. However, 69 percentage of the total children from all villages were immunised for polio, and 41 per cent received injections against measles, and 31 per cent were immunised by a dose of vitamin A against night blindness. But again, it has been noted that village Motipur was poorly covered by immunisation programmes of polio, measles, vitamin A, in addition to BCG and DPT vaccinations. Though, in general the overall immunisation coverage of the children below the age of five years in the study villages does not look poor and discouraging, at individual levels the picture certainly looks quite gloomy for the children in Motipur, followed by the children in Santoshpur.

Although more than one half of the total children were covered by various immunisation services and vaccinations in the study villages, quite a few of the mothers did not take any interest in completing the required vaccine dosage of different vaccinations. The study found that the overall completion rate of DPT vaccination was only 46 per cent. Nearly 44 per cent had taken just one vaccination for DPT instead of the recommended three.

A similar pattern can be observed in case of polio vaccine as well. Most of the infants were not given the recommended three doses of the polio vaccine. A majority of the children were given the polio vaccine much later after birth and 70 per cent of the children had received the complete recommended three doses of the vaccine.

Health Care Utilisation for Children in Case of Illness

During infancy and childhood years very young children often suffer from a wide range of ailments because of exogenous factors, especially from water-borne and air-borne diseases, infections and so on. Most of the surveyed children suffered from some kind of ailment or other during their childhood years. But most of the children suffered from mild fever, flu', cold, cough, dysentery, diarrhoea and other infectious diseases. See table 8.14 for more details.

Table 8.14: **Children ever suffered from illness (0-5 years)**

KIND OF AILMENTS/ILLNESS	MOTIPUR (Tribal, N_1 = 48)	KAPGARI (Hindu, N_2 =68)	SANTOSHPUR (Muslim, N_3 = 54)	SULTANPUR (Developed, N_4 = 31)	TOTAL (N_T = 201)
WHOOPING COUGH	1 (2.08)	6 (8.82%)	5 (9.25%)	2 (6.45%)	14 (6.96%)
MEASLES	11 (22.9%)	10 (14.70%)	15 (27.77%)	18 (58.06%)	54 (26.86%)
MALARIA	3 (6.25%)	-	3 (5.55%)	1 (3.22%)	7 (3.48%)
CHICKEN POX	9 (18.75%)	7 (10.29%)	10 (18.51%)	6 (19.35%)	32 (15.92%)
CHOLERA	1 (2.08)	1 (1.47%)	3 (5.55%)	-	5 (2.48%)
OTHERS (D&D, FEVER, COLD, ETC.)	23 (47.91%)	44 (64.70%)	18 (33.33%)	4 (12.90%)	89 (44.27%)
TOTAL	48 (23.88%)	68 (33.83%)	54 (26.86%)	31 (15.42%)	201

Most of the children suffered from some kind of illness or the other, but a majority of them suffered from dysentery and diarrhoea, fever, cough and cold. Not very many children suffered from any kind of serious ailments besides dysentery and diarrhoea.

Many women did not think it was necessary to seek any treatment for minor illnesses like cough, cold, chicken-pox and measles, for their children. Most of the women said there was no point in seeking treatment for diseases like chicken-pox, measles, and cold, because these ailments take their own time to heal and cure with or without medicines and in the end it cures after a certain length of time. However, almost everyone sought treatment for dysentery, diarrhoea, fever, cholera, malaria, etc. Table 8.15 gives detailed information.

Table 8.15: **Sought treatment for children's illness**

VILLAGE	YES	NO	TOTAL
MOTIPUR (Tribal, N_1 = 48)	30 (62.5%)	18 (37.5%)	48
KAPGARI (Hindu, N_2 = 68)	42 (61.76%)	26 (38.23%)	68
SANTOSHPUR (Muslim, N_3 = 54)	30 (55.55%)	24 (44.44%)	54
SULTANPUR (Developed, N_4 = 31)	20 (64.51%)	11 (35.48%)	31
TOTAL (N_T = 201)	122 (60.69%)	79 (39.30%)	201

It can be seen from the table that overall 61 per cent of the women had sought treatment for their children during illness in their childhood years. However, somewhat fewer women sought treatment for their children during illness in village Santoshpur as opposed to the other study villages. Most of the households in Motipur sought treatment for their children from the public sector and the villagers in Kapgari preferred the private medical sector for treatment for their ill children. The women in Santoshpur also favoured the private medical sector for treatment of their children, though they normally sought and utilised the services of traditional practitioners or homeopathic doctors for very young children. The women in Sultanpur also sought treatment from the private medical sector. Refer to table 8.16 for more information.

Table 8.16:   Kind of treatment sought for children

KIND & TYPE OF TREATMENT SOUGHT	MOTIPUR (Tribal)	KAPGARI (Hindu)	SANTOSHPUR (Muslim)	SULTANPUR (Developed)	TOTAL
PUBLIC SECTOR					
GOVERNMENT /MUNICIPAL HOSPITAL	4 (13.33%)	2 (4.76%)	-	3 (15%)	9 (7.37%)
PRIMARY HEALTH CENTRE (PHC)	15 (50%)	9 (21.42%)	9 (30%)	-	33 (27.04%)
SUB-CENTRE	-	1 (2.38%)	-	-	1 (0.81%)
PRIVATE MEDICAL SECTOR					
PRIVATE HOSPITAL/CLINIC	-	9 (21.42%)	-	1 (5%)	10 (8.19%)
PRIVATE DOCTOR	4 (13.33%)	8 (19.04%)	9 (30%)	7 (35%)	28 (22.95%)
OTHER PRIVATE SECTOR					
TRADITIONAL PRACTITIONER	3 (10%)	5 (11.90%)	5 (16.66%)	4 (20%)	17 (13.93%)
AYURVEDIC DOCTOR	-	-	-	1 (5%)	1 (0.81%)
HOMEOPATHIC DOCTOR	4 (13.33%)	8 (19.04%)	7 (23.33%)	4 (20%)	23 (18.85%)
TOTAL	30 (24.59%)	42 (34.42%)	30 (24.59%)	20 (16.39%)	122

Almost 31 per cent of the total women preferred treatment from the private medical sector and particularly 23 per cent from a private doctor. Twenty-seven per cent sought treatment from the PHCs. Some of the women and their families sought homeopathic treatment for their children in 19 per cent of the cases and 14 per cent relied on the traditional healers and practitioners for treatment of illness during childhood years.

The overall situation reveals that the villagers in Motipur utilise the public sector facilities (63%) much more than the other villages for treatment of their children. In Kapgari, 29 per cent utilise the public sector medical facilities for their children. Thirty per cent utilise public sector medical facilities in Santoshpur compared to only 15 per cent in Sultanpur.

Villages Kapgari, Santoshpur and Sultanpur chose to seek treatment from private doctors because they were economically better off, and could afford to pay the fees of private practitioners. Furthermore, they lacked confidence in the treatment of the doctors in the public medical sectors. The general misconception is that free services are of poorer and lower quality, compared to the private ones.

In case of both males and females during any common ailments like fever, cough, cold, dysentery, diarrhoea, respiratory tract infection, most of the women depending on the type of illness sought treatment. But for very young infants homeopathic treatment was favoured. Furthermore, most of the women said that they preferred to try all types of available remedial treatments.

Normally they first consult with a homeopathic doctor or an ayurvedic doctor for any illness for their children and if the illness persists they then seek treatment from the public medical sector and lastly consult with a private doctor. Whereas in some cases, they first consult with a traditional practitioner and if the problem persists, they then visit a homeopathic doctor for treatment and lastly visit the village PHC or the government hospital for further treatment depending upon the seriousness of the diseases and illness. Refer to table 8.17 for more details.

Table 8.17: **Type of treatment sought for children with common ailments**

TYPE & KIND OF TREATMENT SOUGHT	MOTIPUR	KAPGARI	SANTOSHPUR	SULTANPUR	TOTAL
PRIVATE DOCTOR (ALLOPATHIC)	12 (12.5%)	23 (24.21%)	11 (12.08%)	8 (8.79%)	54 (14.47%)
PRIMARY HEALTH CENTRE (PHC)	70 (72.91%)	40 (42.10%)	43 (47.25%)	34 (37.36%)	187 (50.13%)
FIRST HOMEOPATHY, THEN GOVT. HOSPITAL.	4 (4.16%)	3 (3.15%)	28 (30.76%)	14 (15.38%)	49 (13.13%)
FIRST PHC, THEN PRIVATE DOCTOR	8 (8.33%0	29 (30.52%)	2 (2.19%)	35 (38.46%)	75 (20.10%)
CONSULT TRADITIONAL PRACTITIONER	2 (2.08%)	-	5 (5.49%)	-	7 (1.87%)
NO TREATMENT FOR FEMALES 'COS POOR	-	-	2 (2.19%)	-	2 (0.53%)
TOTAL	96	95	91	91	373
CHILDREN DIED IN INFANCY (N.A.)	**2**	**3**	**1**	**3**	**9**
WOMEN PREGNANT FOR THE FIRST TIME	**4**	**2**	**8**	**6**	**19**

The table shows that almost one half of the total population (50%) visited the PHC along with their infants and children for treatment during any illness. Twenty per cent first went to the PHC, but if the ailment continued they then consulted with any private allopathic practitioners. Only 14 per cent straight away consulted with a private allopathic doctor for treatment of their children in case of any ailments. Overall the population in the study villages normally practised medical pluralism during any kind of illness.

No gender discrimination was found in the treatment of male and female babies. Both were given immediate medical attention and both were taken to all kinds of doctors and practitioners for treatment and cure for any kind of disease and ailment. But medical pluralism exists in all study villages and people have faith in all types of medical and non-medical aspects of treatment and cure.

Though the overall condition of the study villages in terms of immunisation and utilisation of health care for infants and children does not look very dismal, there is a clear-cut difference between the villages in the coverage of its immunisation services and programmes.

Though Motipur is poorly covered by immunisation programmes but they are quite prompt in seeking medical care for their children, both male and female babies. In fact, no gender discrimination was found in the utilisation of health care facilities for infants and children in all villages. A strong belief exists in the study villages that homeopathic medicine is much better for very young infants and children than allopathic medicines, which are too strong for young children. Hence most of the people from all the villages choose more homeopathic treatment for their infants and very young children during any kind of ailment.

Conclusion

The sex ratio at birth was favourable towards male babies, but more male babies died before completing the first year of their life. Breast feeding is universal but is not initiated until after 24 to 72 hours after birth. Time length of breast feeding varied according to the educational attainment of the mothers. The mothers with some schooling introduced supplementary food earlier than the mothers with no schooling. The overall birth weight of an infant was found to be dependent on the socio-economic condition of the household and various maternal factors. No gender discrimination was found in the utilisation of health care facilities for infants and children. However, homeopathic medicines were preferred for infants and very young children during any kind of ailment.

Cultural Dimensions of Women's Health

It is a recognised fact that the health status of the people reflects the socio-economic development of a country and is an indicator of social well-being. Health has also been declared as a fundamental human right. Attainment of health for all has been the central issue and official target of WHO and its member countries to provide an acceptable level of health to all people. Despite these efforts basic health status is not enjoyed by a majority of the people world-wide, particularly, those from the developing countries and especially the poor, urban slum-dwellers and squatters, indigenous people and rural women and men.

In the UN Decade for Women (1975-1985), attention was directed to the issues of women and development. This spurred the establishment of national machinery for the promotion of women's interests where none had existed before. However, the findings suggests that such establishments have achieved little in terms of meeting the health care needs of rural women in India.

As mentioned earlier women in the developing countries often suffer from poor health, but consume less health care as compared to their male counterparts. In addition, they are frequently confronted with numerous socio-cultural factors which affect their overall physiological well-being and their access to appropriate health care services. The findings reiterates this situation. For a woman in the study area, the childbearing years are the most risky, because of poor communication and transportation, lack of adequate safe drinking water and generally low standards of living. Furthermore, the laborious work that women are required to perform has a detrimental effect upon their health, and in certain circumstances, upon the viability of their babies.

Rural Indian women are restricted by and governed by a number of taboos which are generally imposed as a control mechanism. Traditionally taboos range from controlling their movements, decision-making, status within the family, type of clothes they wear, to the food they consume during certain periods of their lives. These taboos and restrictions still hold true in most rural areas of the country, and the majority of rural women strictly adhere to

183

these taboos, particularly during pregnancy, lactation, and after delivery. Taboos are handed down through the generations as a collective consciousness of the society. They are a set of norms which are believed to be an effective system for coping with the uncertainty of nature. Social policies need to be developed to attack the assumptions behind taboos which are against the best interests of women and children.

Health Care Infrastructure

India adopted the National Health Policy (NHP) in June 1981 and this was approved by the Parliament in 1983. The delivery of health services is mainly governed by the National Health Policy which places a major emphasis on ensuring primary health care to all by the year 2000. The NHP identifies certain areas which need special attention and they are: (1) nutrition for all segments of the population, (2) immunisation programme, (3) maternal and child health care, (4) prevention of food adulteration and maintenance of the quality of drugs, (5) water supply and sanitation, (6) environmental protection, (7) school health programmes, (8) occupational health services, and (9) prevention and control of locally endemic diseases (IIPS, 1995). After the Alma Ata Declaration in 1978, government of India began developing the rural health infrastructure to provide health care services to the rural population which had been largely neglected earlier in order to move towards the goal of "Health for All" by 2000 AD.

State Level Health Infrastructure

Since the delivery of health services is mainly governed by the NHP, the health policies are formulated at the centre. The allocation of resources for health services to the states are also controlled by the central government. However, as health is seen as a state subject under the Indian Constitution, the responsibility for providing health services are with the State Department of Health and Family Welfare of each state (Kannan et al., 1991). The State Department of Health and Family Welfare is headed by a minister and an administrative officer (IAS), who serves as the secretary in-charge of administration. In addition, there are state directorates of health and family welfare represented by a director of health services, and under this are the additional, deputy and assistant director for individual programmes like immunisation, family planning, maternal and child health, etc.

District Level Health Infrastructure

At the district level, the health services structure and organisation varies from state to state. But the overall structure of the district is under the control of District Medical/Health Officer, who is assisted by two deputy district medical officers. In most of the states, all the districts have district hospitals where curative services are provided. In the district hospitals, specialist care like paediatrics, ophthalmology, ENT, obstetrics and gynaecology, general surgery and general medicines are available.

Rural Health Infrastructure

The Primary Health Centre (PHC) is the core institution of the rural health services infrastructure in India. According to the present infrastructure, there is one sub-centre for every 5,000 population, one PHC for every 30,000 population and one Community Health Centre (CHC) for every 100,000 - 120,000 population. In tribal and hilly areas, one sub-centre is planned for every 3,000 population and one PHC for every 20,000 population. As of March 1992, there were 20,719 PHCs and 131,464 sub-centres, providing health and family welfare services to the rural population (Government of India, 1994).

At the PHC, two or three Medical Officers are assisted by a paramedical staff of 15 to 20 persons, including Public Health Nurses (PHNs), Lady Health Visitors (LHVs), Block Extension Educators (BEEs), and so on, to provide both centre-based and outreach services to the villages in their jurisdiction. The PHCs are to have specialist facilities in obstetrics and gynaecology, paediatrics, etc., but most PHCs do not have any of these facilities in most states. The system of specialist care extends upwards to secondary and tertiary facilities in the form of District and Sub-Divisional hospitals and larger municipal hospitals in the cities (Bhende and Kanitkar, 1993; Kannan et al., 1991; Chatterjee, 1990).

The rural health system at present offers family welfare services, including maternal and child health schemes through the network of PHCs, sub-centres, and referral centres called the Community Health Centres (CHCs), and also through the Village Health Guides (VHGs) and Traditional Birth

Attendants (TBAs) at the village level. Furthermore, the National Child Survival and Safe Motherhood (CSSM) Programme provides a package of services combining immunisation with maternal and child health care interventions (Ministry of Health and Family Welfare, 1992).

In the establishment of this health system, the major strategies for the provision of MCH services have been: (1) the training of ANMs and their deployment at health centres; (2) provision of specialised medical services in obstetrics and gynaecology at the PHCs, including one female Medical Officer and two certified nurses; (3) establishment of maternity beds in hospitals at all levels; and (4) training of village *dais* and VHGs to provide domiciliary services (Chatterjee, 1990).

The National Health Policy Goals

The long term and major national demographic goal is to achieve replacement-level fertility (Net Reproduction Rate of 1.0) by 2016. As part of this goal, the country aims to reduce the crude birth rate to 21 per 1,000, the crude death rate to 9 per 1,000, and the infant mortality rate to below 60 per 1,000 live births, and to increase the effective couple protection rate (the percentage of eligible couples effectively protected through any family planning method) to 60 per cent. In addition, the National Child Survival and Safe Motherhood Programme has introduced additional health goals. The programme aims to reduce infant mortality to 50 by 2000, reduce the child mortality rate (at ages 1-4) from 41 to less than 10 by 2000, eliminate tetanus among neonates by 1995, prevent 95 per cent of deaths due to measles and reduce measles cases by 90 per cent, prevent 70 per cent of deaths due to diarrhoea and reduce diarrhoea cases by 25 per cent and prevent 40 per cent of deaths due to acute respiratory infection by 2000 (Ministry of Health and Family Welfare, 1992). It is indeed unfortunate that none of these goals have still been achieved and there are no indication of its accomplishment in the very near future too.

In India, MCH and family planning services are integrated within the family welfare programme, and the focus of this programme has been on numbers rather than on the quality of services to women's health needs. The result is that the quality of services is severely compromised and achievement of demographic targets has taken precedence over individual concerns. Because of this narrow focus of the current family welfare programme, it has had limited success in achieving even its limited objectives of reducing birth rates and improving maternal and child health. To what extent the country will be successful in achieving the targets laid down with respect to various health indicators remains to be seen given the current emphasis on numbers rather than the overall health needs of women.

Fundamental Shortcomings

The National Health Policy recognises the failure of the existing health system to reach women, especially in the rural areas, but still does not specifically discuss women's health issues, nor recognises the importance of improving women's health. Problems of implementation have hampered the effectiveness of the pyramidal health structure and policy which has been established both in the rural and the urban areas.

As health services fall under the dual responsibility of the central and the state governments, the state government receives only a fragment of the total health care budget of the centre, and the rest comes from the states own budget. However, certain health policies formulated by the central government are totally under their directive like the family planning programme, immunisation coverage programme, nutritional programmes, maternal and child health care services and eradication of diseases like the measles, polio, night blindness, etc. The centre allocates only a portion of the total national health budget to the state governments. The most populous states in the country and the larger states receive more resources for health services from the centre and allocation is primarily determined on the basis of population size of the state and its total area. However, in reality more budget is usually allocated to the states with the same ruling party in power both at the centre and at the state level. This brings about uneven development between the states and also at the rural and urban levels as more budget is allocated for the urban centres and large cities as opposed to the rural areas.

The major responsibility of the state government therefore is to oversee the administration of state run hospitals, PHCs, and other clinics and hospitals and maintain its expenditure. Since a majority of the programmes related to women's health are implemented directly from the centre, the state government ensures its administration and cost-effective maintenance at the state level. The state appoints a director of health services who is responsible for the implementation of the various programmes at the district level, sub-division and village level with the help of additional deputy directors.

Hence, the NHP's aims to rectify the problem via extensive primary health care approach, with special attention to maternal and child health services, nutrition and immunisation programmes has not been very successful at the grassroots level. This is because of a highly centralised structure, where monitoring of health personnel and implementation of services, co-ordination between the different tiers of health services becomes immensely difficult because of lack of communication facilities and geographical locations. Moreover, the health staff at the PHC level are more involved with achieving family planning targets, as failure to do so is punishable. Further, the doctors are not greatly motivated, dedicated nor committed to their jobs and are very reluctant to work in the rural areas because of lack of basic facilities and infrastructure like accommodation, potable water, sanitation, electricity, etc. The doctors are forcibly assigned against their wish to serve in the rural health centres for a period of two years immediately upon their graduation because of a strict government stipulation (the government's approach in providing primary health care to the rural people). Because of these factors the doctors are not always present, or if they are present, they do not take their work seriously, instead, concentrate more on their private practice to earn more money. The government should at least provide basic infrastructure before assigning doctors to the rural areas. As an added incentive it should make provision to pay more to the doctors willing to work in the rural areas, and increase their non-practice allowance. In addition, the health personnel should be provided with easy communication facilities and transportation to enable them to monitor and implement and co-ordinate various programmes at the grassroots level in their jurisdiction.

Barriers to Women's Health

MCH in India has received considerable attention because of the need to reduce excess mortality and morbidity among mothers and children and has been incorporated at all levels of health policy. Despite the primary health care approach, major deficiency in service delivery have prevented the health system from dealing successfully with women's health issues.

Critical Problems of Service Delivery

At the village level, Volunteer Health Guides (VHGs) have been entrusted with providing basic treatment of common ailments, health education, and simple disease control measures like chlorinating drinking water sources. The

VHG scheme has been limited in its ability to reach women because of the failure to recruit female VHGs in most states. In addition, they are paid only a token honorarium and, hence, do not take their work seriously. For extensive coverage of out-reach services at the village level, it is imperative to recruit staff. Besides, incentives in the form of improved wages, transportation should be arranged for the staff to take their work seriously and for extensive coverage in the villages under their jurisdiction.

The trained *dai* scheme has fallen short of expectations despite its extensive coverage. This is because of the low social status of *dais* in Indian society, where they are regarded primarily as sweepers who clean up after childbirth. This has denied them the potential of becoming true community health workers. Besides, the quality (and quantity) of their training and support is also inadequate. The Traditional Birth Attendants (TBAs) are trained to provide prenatal and postnatal care and to conduct modern, aseptic deliveries (by using pre-packed sterile delivery kits) and are to provide referral services to the next level. But this has been unsuccessful because of the traditional beliefs and practices surrounding childbirth. Innovations such as the provision of safe delivery kits to mothers has been successful in certain areas, where at the time of delivery, even if a *dai* is present or not, the umbilical cord can be cleanly cut and cared for, in order to reduce the risks of neonatal tetanus. The other is the provision of additional incentive money to *dais* to attend and report births.

The female health workers, or Auxiliary Nurse Midwives (ANMs), provide maternal and child health and family planning services to women. It is intended that 90 per cent of the health problems are to be dealt with at this or below this level, the remaining being referred to the PHCs. MCH services are also rendered at the village level by trained Anganwadi Workers (AWWs), together with the health staff under the Integrated Child Development Services (ICDS) Scheme. ICDS combines basic health care with supplementary nutrition for children and pregnant or lactating women and pre-school education services.

Although the ANM is the key women's health functionary, many problems hamper her effectiveness. Inadequate facilities and other social/personal problems dissuade ANMs from residing at their village headquarters and they are not always available to women when they are needed. In their outreach mode, they are unable to cover their target populations with the range of services entrusted to them because of geography and other reasons. In addition, there is a shortage of ANMs in most states. Moreover their wages are low and working conditions are poor. ANMs remain professionally underdeveloped for lack of adequate in-service training and supervision. The problem of low pay and low status affect the female health workers motivation and morale. Further there is a need for improvement in the wages, transportation, communication, accommodation, safety and proper infrastructure to recruit more female health workers. In addition, ANMs, as well as other female health workers, require psychological and motivational support. If the ANMs could also be locally recruited the problem of accommodation, safety and security would be ensured and they would then reside in their village headquarters itself and would be available to women at all times.

One of the foremost problems faced by ANM's MCH work is the health system's emphasis on workers having to meet family planning targets (so that higher-level facilities can in turn meet theirs, for example, PHCs, District Health/Medical Officers, etc.). The fact that failure to do so is punishable, results in little MCH work being done. There are neither incentives nor penalties and no targets associated for MCH work. Furthermore, it is essential to staff the health centres with ANMs trained and equipped to handle women's health complaints, and deploy them to provide paramedical services regularly at the village level, as this is the most important level of health care provision for rural women. However, the full potential of ANMs can only be realised through vastly improved training and methodical support. In particular, ANMs must be encouraged to pay attention to women's health, and not just family planning.

Key Findings

This study explored the health of women in rural India in the age group of 13-49 years. It primarily explored the maternal and child health care practices in rural West Bengal state, with an emphasis on women's reproductive health, family planning, health care behaviour and utilisation of health care services. The key findings indicates certain similarities and differences in health care behaviour between the villages. However, the strong influence of culture and tradition on certain aspects of health care behaviour was observed in all the villages. Services provided by primary health care seems to have a limited impact on the study population. Some of the key issues are reiterated here.

Similarities in Health Care Utilisation and Behaviour

Medical pluralism was found to be flourishing and more than one medical system was used simultaneously to cure an ailment because health care behaviour in rural India is almost invariably flexible, and people switch from one medical system to another depending on affordability and time. Sometimes they even utilise the services of more than one practitioner simultaneously (Beals, 1976; Leslie, 1976; Jeffrey, 1988; Kakar *et al.*, 1972; Kamat, 1995). Health and welfare policy makers should take into consideration the strong belief of the local population in the Indian systems of medicine, especially for the treatment of very young children.

Even though MCH programmes are implemented in the villages through the PHCs, the concept of "postnatal care" is almost non-existent in the study villages. A policy and programme initiative is required to promote postnatal care vigorously; its benefits and importance both for the health of the mother and the child are very great.

Very few women registered for a postnatal check-up. This low percentage of postnatal clinic attendance is due to the compulsory confinement of the mother and the new-born for a certain period of time after delivery. Further, women thought postnatal care was not at all necessary. Besides, they had no knowledge about postnatal clinics. Low level of utilisation of postnatal services is because of the fact that postnatal health care have not been widely publicised in the country and even the health staff and personnel do not emphasise the need for such care. Therefore, there is a need to publicise and campaign more about postnatal health care in the rural areas of the country to make women aware of the benefits of postnatal care both for the mother and the child and should be made available at homes.

One of the significant achievements of the PHCs is the coverage of immunisation services for children. Most of the children were immunised against tuberculosis, tetanus, whooping cough and polio.

Disparity in Health Care

Access to health care is mediated by several factors other than the health care needs of the mothers. The socio-economic condition of the household, availability of communication and transportation, time constraints, etc. override the health needs. The best levels of utilisation of health care services for family planning, maternal and child health care, labour and delivery were observed in the socio-economically developed village as opposed to the other villages.

Influence of Culture and Tradition

Tradition and culture is often perceived to conspire against well-being, but culture also plays a positive role in certain areas, and breast feeding is one of them. Breast feeding was found to be universal, intensive and prolonged, because of its contraceptive capacity and also because breast milk is best for the child.

Culture and tradition was found to influence age at marriage and age at first birth which is very low at present; and belief in pollution after childbirth and food taboos and practices after delivery and during lactation are followed because of culture and tradition.

'Culture of son preference' is strong and is entwined with the age old tradition of patriarchy.

Policy and programme initiatives should be culturally sensitive and should keep in mind the positive and negative influence of traditional values and norms while formulating programmes for the rural masses.

Limited Impact of PHC

A limited impact of primary health care was observed in the study villages. This is basically due to culturally insensitive service delivery, inadequate and/ or non-availability of medicines and medical facilities, inadequate staffing and non-professional attitudes of staff, long waiting time and unsuitable opening hours of the health centres. Urgent policy and programme initiatives are needed to make PHCs respond more responsibly to the health needs of the women in rural areas.

Socio-Economic Factors

Socio-economic factors affect both a mother's and her children's health which further worsens because of the environmental and hygienic factors like unclean water and food; unsanitary disposal of waste; water-borne disease (diarrhoea, dysentery, cholera, etc.), air-borne diseases like respiratory tract infection, and fever (Chen et al., 1981). The study confirms that social factors such as condition of the house, toilet facilities, crowding, quality of drinking water, source of fuel, lighting; taboos; poverty; ignorance, lack of education of the mother, religion, caste, tribe, so on, also affect the health status of a family. The programme and policy challenge will be to consolidate the socio-economic factors which affect women's health with the overall structure of health care delivery system in the rural areas.

Immediate Factors

As mentioned earlier socio-economic factors affect a mother's and her children's health both directly and indirectly. These indirect socio-economic factors influence women's health through certain immediate factors like the health and nutritional status of the mother; reproductive status; utilisation of health services and health care behaviour, preference for male children, family planning, prenatal care, home deliveries, etc.

Cultural Practices

The literature shows that in many traditional societies of the world, death, birth and other personal and family events entail danger and lead to the seclusion of affected persons, to prohibitions against contact and avoidance of certain foods or actions. In India persons affected in this way are impure for a period of time. Though childbirth is a joyous occasion in almost all parts of the country, nevertheless, it is regarded as impure and polluting, particularly for the mother and the new-born. Therefore, to prevent the entire household from being polluted and impure, normally the mother and the baby are kept away from the main house for a certain period of time.

This polluting factor was very much in evidence in the study population, particularly after childbirth, and the period of seclusion depends on a number of factors, like, caste and religion. Nowadays it also depends on the economic value and contribution of the mother towards the household income. Hence, depending on the caste, religion, socio-economic and socio-cultural backgrounds, and social standing of the household in the community, the period of isolation varies. Strict food taboos are imposed on women immediately after delivery and most women in the study population strictly adhere to them irrespective of religion, caste, geographical location and so on.

Restrictive diet is given to the mothers immediately after childbirth and this diet continues till the woman is in seclusion. After that she is allowed to eat normally, but again, depending on the health and condition of the child the diet is changed constantly.

The study population strongly believes in the theory of pollution and impurity after childbirth. An appropriate health education strategy is important and necessary in enhancing and maintaining the quality of maternal health in the context of cultural practices associated with child birth and lactation. Programmes should take into consideration the sensitive issue of pollution and impurity and formulate programmes to provide nutritional supplements and postnatal care to mothers at home by the health staff.

Breast Feeding

Most of the women avoid certain food, which according to them, are harmful for the infant. The foodstuffs avoided during the initial stages of lactation vary with age, religion, caste, economic status, and also vary from place to place producing distinct dietary patterns. They normally avoid food which according to them, has laxative properties or food considered to be cold, or food that could cause skin rash and also avoid food which they consider to be acidic. These foodstuffs are avoided in the best interest of the child to whom harmful elements could be passed through mother's milk. Different social groups and communities have different norms and practices that they follow during lactation.

The food taboos and avoidance imposed on women during any period of their life are justified to be in the best interest of both the women and their infants, and to protect them from any kind and type of impairment and ill health. Nevertheless, the taboos, prejudices and beliefs and attitudes centring around food are cultural practices that act as blocks preventing full utilisation of the available food during postpartum period when it is most essential.

Specific Recommendations

The health sector needs to concentrate on improving the availability of affordable and cost-effective health services by:

a) Improving village-level health care activities carried out by *dais*, VHGs and AWWs, and extending these to encompass women's basic health needs like distribution of iron-folate supplements, in addition to antenatal care, birth attendance, postnatal care and child care services.

b) Strengthening MCH care at PHCs to cater to the health needs of women and children, making services readily available to them, and co-ordinating basic health care with preventive measures such as immunisation and nutrition improvement. There is a need to develop an efficient referral system from village to sub-centre to PHC and beyond. Greater attention should be paid to strengthening the lower levels of the health systems.

c) Increased allocations will be necessary to ensure adequate provisions for personnel, their training and better administration and supervision. A larger

MCH budget within the general health and family welfare budget should be earmarked separately by the state governments as well.

d) Although designed to cater to pregnant and nursing women, national nutrition programmes fail to induce women to attend - mainly because they ignore the social strictures against women eating in public, their need/inclination to share food with other household members, their lack of time, etc. Women who do attend supplementary feeding programmes may be denied their household share of food. Thus, the mechanics of supplementary feeding schemes must pay greater attention to the household situation, if pregnant women are to receive even the very small supplement of 500 calories envisioned for them (Chatterjee, 1990). Therefore greater emphasis on women's nutritional supplementation, health care and health-nutrition education is required, with time set aside by workers specifically to motivate and cater to women (through home visits), particularly those in low-income families.

e) Investment in primary education is the most effective way to reduce fertility in the long term and the family welfare programme should reorient towards birth-spacing methods rather than sterilisation.

f) Regional differences in manpower and services availability need to be addressed, particularly the lack of women doctors. While some rural women will approach male doctors for general complaints, the examination or treatment of gynaecological or obstetric problems require the presence of a woman doctor. Thus, with the lack of lady doctors at the PHC level, most women-specific diseases are neglected.

g) The major responsibility of the health system lies in extending availability. Outreach workers fail to reach into homes, to overcome the constraints of lack of permission facing most rural women, and to impart preventive and promotive health care. Since institution-based care currently remains inaccessible to the majority of women and children and since the purpose of outreach schemes is specifically to overcome the constraints faced by women in approaching (socially or physically) health centres, these workers must be deployed in such a way as to provide services "at the doorstep".

h) The location, nature and quality of services must be made proportionate with existing health problems and needs. In order to make the system more responsive to women's needs, it is necessary to gather information on the general health problems of women, other women-specific health problems, women's utilisation of health services, and women's attitudes to health problems and services through community-wide surveys.

i)   There have not been adequate efforts to improve awareness of health services and to create demand for them through information and education. Little knowledge exists of preventive services and health education is rarely taken seriously by the providers or the clients. The public must be educated about health and disease and about prevention and treatment, especially of women's problems, in order for services to become accessible to them. The problem of availability can be tackled by increasing health services that cater to women's health needs, providing these services at locations where women can utilise them at all times and improving the quality of these services. In addition women need to be empowered to demand for services essential to them. This can be achieved by bringing about a change in their perception and attitude towards their own health with the help of education which in turn will enhance knowledge and awareness about health and health services, thereby, increasing demand for better service delivery.

j)   The attitudes of service providers and policy-makers towards women require considerable change. Women's health has been regarded as a welfare issue and their economic roles have been largely ignored and inadequate attention has been paid even to their roles as unpaid domestic workers. Because of long waiting time at the health centres and inadequate attention to women, greatly increases the opportunity costs of seeking health care and therefore they are discouraged from doing so. Routine visits of outreach workers also often fail to take into account the fact that their clients may be out to work - so that coverage is further reduced. The opportunity costs of obtaining health care for women can be reduced, for instance, by ensuring more efficient provision of services so that time is not wasted at health centres; by ensuring that wages are not lost while health care is sought/obtained. If services are made available closer to homes little money is spent travelling to health centres; and so on.

k)   In fact, increasing women's access to health services is critical for the achievement of the postulated mortality, morbidity and fertility reduction goals, and in addition, the National Health Policy's primary health care approach require a woman-centred perspective towards health care delivery system.

However, active community participation, deployment of dedicated paramedical health staff at the village level and willing doctors, nurses and other health personnel at the PHC level seems to be of utmost importance for successful implementation of health programmes in the rural areas of the country. India is still far from reaching the ideal of Health for All by 2000 AD, is because of its narrow focus and emphasis on meeting targets and numbers rather than addressing the overall issue of women's reproductive health needs.

Summary

The framework adopted for the present study from McCarthy and Maine (1993) is appropriate and useful in exploring and presenting the health condition of rural women and children in West Bengal. However, one of the limitations of the McCarthy and Maine model is that they have consolidated the socio-economic and cultural factors, and have given less importance to the cultural factors contributing towards maternal health and morbidity. The revised framework by the researcher illustrates cultural factors to greatly influence the outcome of mother's health status in rural India. Because the cultural factors associated with pregnancy, labour and delivery, and lactation play a major role and is an immediate determinant affecting maternal health in rural India. Hence the revised framework has been found to be adequate in exploring and understanding MCH in rural India. The framework can be useful in formulation of policy and programmes and can be used for programme evaluation and analyses. The modified framework can be further revised for further research in maternal and child health care in rural area.

Overall the study found a significant link between socio-economic development, particularly women's development, and health care behaviour and utilisation. Socio-economic development was found to change people's view towards health and transformed their orientation towards better health care and maximum utilisation of the available health care services. Furthermore, socio-economic status and religion was found to play a crucial role in influencing all the variables in the study and illustrates the significance of socio-economic development and health care behaviour. The key findings suggests some similarities and differences in health care behaviour between the villages. Culture, religion and tradition, have an impact on certain aspects of health care utilisation and behaviour. Furthermore, the study observed the services of the primary health care centres to have limited impact.

The study found religious beliefs and ethnicity play an important role in utilisation of health services. It has been noted that registration and attendance at antenatal clinics were high, but registration and attendance at postnatal clinics was almost non-existent. Differences in health care behaviour were observed, particularly with regards to labour and delivery. However, irrespective of socio-economic development, belief in pollution after childbirth was strong and culture played a dominant role in practices and taboos observed after childbirth and during lactation. Breast feeding was universal, intensive, and prolonged without any adequate supplementary diet. Age at betrothal and marriage was found to be low irrespective of religious beliefs, caste or socio-economic development.

Hence it can be said that tradition and culture play a much more dominant role with regards age at marriage, practices and taboos observed after delivery and during lactation. Though family planning acceptance was high amongst the educated and socio-economically developed, the small family norm message does not seem to have penetrated in the rural areas.

Medical pluralism was much in evidence in the study villages and more than one medical system was used simultaneously by the surveyed population depending on the perceived severity of illness. A further finding indicates 'consumer oriented' health care behaviour for perceived major ailments and 'welfare oriented' behaviour for perceived minor ailments. Depending on the perceived severity of illness the study population oscillated between either 'consumer oriented' or 'welfare oriented' health care utilisation. Immunisation services and facilities are widely used in the study villages irrespective of religion, caste, geographical location or socio-economic development.

The findings reveal utilisation of health care services for male and female children operated in a unique pattern. For male children homeopathic treatment was preferred and for female children allopathic treatment was sought because of the belief that allopathic medicines are too strong for sons. But sex discrimination in terms of breast feeding, or in health care behaviour was not found despite son preference. This can be understood in the wider socio-cultural context of West Bengal where there is less discrimination against female children, unlike the northern parts of the country.

The study confirms that socio-economic development plays an important role in changing the attitudes and behaviour of the population and enhances their knowledge and awareness about the modern health services and increases its utilisation. Irrespective of socio-economic development and religion, culture and tradition control most women's movement; they are not allowed to move anywhere without being accompanied by a male relative. However, with increasing socio-economic status the hold of religion, tradition and culture begins to slacken, as noted in the developed village where the Muslim women's health care behaviour is unlike that of the women from the Muslim village and is very similar to that of the other women from the developed village.

Undoubtedly socio-economic development and women's education are the determinant factors in changing health care attitudes and increasing utilisation of modern health care services. Yet an appropriate policy and programme framework for addressing the comprehensive health care needs of rural women, particularly of maternal and child health is needed. Immediate political commitment is needed to address the gap between the urban and rural areas of the country in achieving the goal of health for all by the year 2000.

Bibliography

Acsadi, G. T. and Johnson-Acsadi, G., 1991. "Social and Cultural Factors Influencing Maternal and Child Mortality in Sub-Saharan Africa". *The Effects of Maternal Mortality on Children in Africa*, Defense for Children International-USA.

Acsadi, G. T., and Johnson-Acsadi, G., 1986. *Optimum Demographic Conditions of Childbearing*. London, International Planned Parenthood Federation.

Acsadi, George T. and G. Johnson-Acsadi, 1990. "Demand For Children and Child spacing". Chapter 11 in: *Population Growth and Reproduction in Sub-Saharan Africa: Technical Analyses of Fertility and its Consequences*, George T. F. Acsadi, G. Johnson-Acsadi, and Rodolfo A. Bulatao (eds.), Washington, DC, The World Bank.

Akhtar Rais, Learmouth, A. T. A., 1986 (eds.). *Geographical Aspects of Health and Disease in India*, New Delhi, Concept Publishing Co.

Alauddin, M., 1986. "Maternal Mortality in Bangladesh: The Tangail District". *Studies in Family Planning*, Vol. 17, pp. 13-22.

Armstrong, A., 1987. *Women and Law in Southern Africa*. Harare, Zimbabwe Publishing House.

Atal, Y., 1978. "Continuity and Change in a Complex Society: Caste Hierarchy in a Madhya Pradesh Village". *Eastern Anthropologist*, Vol. 31, No. 1, pp. 41-63.

Babbie, E., 1992 (6th ed.). *The Practice of Social Research*. Belmont, California, Wadsworth Publishing Company.

Balzer, M. M., 1981. "Rituals of Gender Identity: Markers of Siberian Khanty Ethnicity, Status, and Belief". *American Anthropologist*, Vol. 83, No. 4, pp. 850-867.

Banerji, D., 1975. "Social and Cultural Foundations of the Health Services Systems in India". *Comparative Health Systems. Supplement to Inquiry*, Vol. 12, pp. 70.

Banerji, D., 1973. "Health Behaviour of Rural Populations: Impact of Rural Health Services". *Economic and Political Weekly*, Vol. 8, No. 51, pp. 2261.

Banerji, D., 1981. "The Place of Indigenous and Western Systems of Medicine in the Health Services of India". *Social Science and Medicine*, Vol. 15A, March, pp. 109-114.

Basu, A. M., 1987. "Household Influences on Child Mortality: The Evidence from Mortality Trends". *Social Biology*, Vol. 34, No. 3-4, pp. 187- 205.

Basu, A. M., 1989a. *Cultural Differences in the Status of Women in India*. Population Transition in India, Monograph prepared for the 21st IUSSP Conference, A. Bose and P. B. Desai (eds.), New Delhi, B. R. Publishing Corporation.

Basu, A. M., 1989b. "Is Discrimination in Food Really Necessary for Explaining Sex Differentials in Childhood Mortality?" *Population Studies*, Vol. 43, No. 2, pp. 193-210.

Basu, A. M., 1989c. "Nutritional Discrimination and Child Mortality". *Population Studies*, Vol. 43, No. 2, pp. 193-210.

Basu, A. M., 1990. "Cultural Influences on Health Care Use: Two Regional Groups in India". *Studies in Family Planning*, Vol. 21, No. 5, pp. 275-286.

Bauer, D. F., and Karp, I., 1978. *Ritual Aspects of Medical Practice*. Pennsylvania Association of Sociological Society (PASS), Paper.

Beals, A. R., 1976. "Strategies of Resort to Cures in South India". *Asian Medical Systems*, Berkeley, University of California Press. pp. 184-200

Beenstock, M. and Sturdy, P., 1990. "The Determinants of Infant Mortality in Regional India". *World Development*, Vol. 8, No. 3, pp. 443-453.

Belsey, M. A., and Royston, E., 1987. *Overview of the Health of Women and Children*. New York, Population Council.

Bergesen, A. J., 1978. "Review Essay: Rituals, Symbols, and Society—Explicating the Mechanisms of the Moral Order". *American Journal of Sociology*, Vol. 83, No. 4, pp. 1012-1021.

Bhatia, J. C., 1973. "Abortionists and Abortion Seekers". *Indian Journal of Social Work*, Vol. 34, No. 3, pp. 275-285.

Bhatia, J. C., 1982a. *Evaluation of Traditional Birth Attendants (DAIS) Training Scheme in the State of Karnataka*. Bangalore, Indian Institute of Management. Unpublished.

Bhatia, J. C., 1982b. *Evaluation of Traditional Birth Attendants (DAIS) Training Scheme in the State of Maharashtra*. Bangalore, Indian Institute of Management. Unpublished.

Bhatia, J. C., 1985. "Impact of Training on the Performance of Traditional Birth Attendants: A Study in Maharashtra State". *Journal of Family Welfare*, Vol. 32, No. 3, pp. 50-61.

Bhatia, J. C., 1986. *A Study of Maternal Mortality in Anantpur District, Andhra Pradesh, India*. Bangalore, Indian Institute of Management.

Bhatia, J. C., 1993. "Levels and Causes of Maternal Mortality in Southern India". *Studies in Family Planning*, Vol. 24, No. 5, pp. 310-318.

Bhatia, J. C., and Mehta, S. R., 1972. "Induced Abortions: Opinions of Indigenous Medicine Practitioners". *Indian Journal of Social Work*, Vol. 32, No. 4, pp. 435-443.

Bhende, A. A., and Kanitaker, T., 1993. *Principles of Population Studies*. Bombay, Himalaya Publishing House.

Bitran, R., 1988. *Health Care Demand Studies in the Developing Countries: A Critical Review and Agenda for Research*. Resources for Child Health Project, Washington, DC, 1988.

Blalock, H. M., 1972 (2nd ed.). *Social Statistics*. New York, McGraw-Hill Ltd.

Blanchet, T., 1984. *Meanings and Rituals of Birth in Rural Bangladesh*. Bangladesh,

Dhaka University Press.

Booth, B. E., and Verma, M., 1992. "Decreased Access to Medical Care for Girls in Punjab, India: The Role of Age, Religion, and Distance". *American Journal of Public Health*, Vol. 82, No. 8, pp. 1155-1157.

Bose, A., 1987. "For Whom the Target Tolls: A Critique of Family Planning Incentives, Cash Awards and Targets". Presidential Address to the 12th Annual Conference of the Indian Association for the Study of Population, Allahabad, India.

Cain, M., 1984. *Women's Status and Fertility in Developing Countries: Son Preference and Economic Security*, World Bank Staff Working Paper no. 682. Washington, DC, The World Bank.

Caldwell P. and Caldwell, J. C., 1987. "Where There is a Narrower Gap Between Female and Male Situations: Lessons From South India and Sri Lanka". Paper Presented at the Social Science Research Council Workshop on Gender Differentials in Mortality in South Asia, Dhaka, Bangladesh.

Caldwell, J. C., 1979. "Education as a Factor in Mortality Decline: An Examination of Nigerian data". *Population Studies*, Vol. 33, No. 3, pp. 395-413.

Caldwell, J. C., 1986. "Routes to Low Mortality in Poor Countries". *Population and Development Review*, Vol. 12, No. 2, pp. 171-220.

Caldwell, J. C., 1989. "Mass Education as a Determinant of Mortality Decline". *Cultural, Social and Behavioural Determinants of Health*, John C. Caldwell and Gigi Santow (eds.), Canberra, Australian National University, Health Transition Centre, pp. 103-111.

Caldwell, J. C., 1990. "Cultural and Social Factors Influencing Mortality Levels in Developing Countries". *Annals of the American Academy of Political and Social Science*, Vol. 510, pp. 44-59.

Caldwell, J. C., and Caldwell, P., 1990. "Cultural Forces Tending to Sustain High Fertility". Chapter 13 in: *Population Growth and Reproduction in Sub-Saharan Africa: Technical Analyses of Fertility and its Consequences*. George T. F. Acsadi, G. Johnson-Acsadi, and Rodolfo A. Bulatao (eds.), Washington, DC, The World Bank.

Caldwell, J. C., and McDonald, P., 1982. "Influence of Maternal Education on Infant and Child Mortality: Levels and Causes". *Proceedings of IUSSP Conference in Manila*, Vol. 2, pp. 79-95.

Caldwell, J. C., Reddy, P. H., and Caldwell, P., 1983. "The Social Component of Mortality Decline: An Investigation in South India Employing Alternative Methodologies". *Population Studies*, Vol. 37, No. 2, pp. 185-206.

Cancellier, P. H., and Crews, K. A., 1986. *Women in the World: The Women's Decade and Beyond*. Washington, DC, Population Reference Bureau.

Cassen, R. H., 1982. *India: Population, Economy, Society*. London, MacMillan.

Chatterjee, M., 1985. "Women's Access to Health Services". In Proceedings of *Workshop on Child Health, Nutrition and Family Planning*, November 1983, New Delhi, Indian Council of Medical Research.

Chatterjee, M., 1990. *Indian Women: Their Health and Economic Productivity*. World

Bank Discussion Papers:109, Washington DC, The World Bank.

Chaudhuri, B., 1986. *Tribal Studies of India Series T 120: Tribal Health æ Sociocultural Dimensions*, New Delhi, Inter-India Publications.

Chavkin W., and St Clain D., 1990. "Beyond Prenatal Care: A Comprehensive Vision of Reproductive Health". *Journal of American Med. Women Assoc.* Vol. 45, No. 2, pp. 55-57.

Chen, L. C., Huq, E., and D'Souza, S., 1981. "Sex Bias in the Family Allocation of Food and Health Care in Rural Bangladesh". *Population and Development Review*, Vol. 7, No. 1, pp. 55-70.

Clark, A. W., 1987. "Social Demography of Excess Female Mortality in India: New Directions". *Economic and Political Weekly*, Vol. 22, No. 17, pp. WS-12.

Cleland J., 1989. "Maternal Education and Child Survival: Further Evidence and Explanations". *What We Know About Health Transition: The Proceedings of an International Workshop*, John C. Caldwell et al. (eds.), Canberra, May 1989, Australian National University, Health Transition Centre.

Cleland, J. G., and Sathar, Z. A., 1984. "The Effect of Birth Spacing on Childhood Mortality in Pakistan". *Population Studies*, Vol. 38, pp. 402-408.

Cochrane, S. H., 1979. *Fertility and Education: What Do We Really Know?* Baltimore, MD, Johns Hopkins University Press.

Curtin, L. B., 1982. *Status of Women: A Comparative Analysis of Twenty Developing Countries*. Monograph. Reports on the World Fertility Survey, 5 (AID/DSPE-C-0024).

D'Souza, S., and Lincoln C., 1980. "Sex Differentials in Mortality in Rural Bangladesh". *Population and Development Review*, Vol. 6, No. 2, pp. 257-270.

Das Gupta, M., 1987. "Selective Discrimination Against Female Children in Rural Punjab, India". *Population and Development Review*, Vol. 13, No. 1, pp. 77-100.

Das Gupta, M., 1989. "The Effects of Discrimination on Health and Mortality". Proceedings of the *International Union for the Scientific Study of Population* (IUSSP), New Delhi, International Population Conference.

Das Gupta, M., 1990. "Death Clustering, Mother's Education and the Determinants of Child Mortality in Rural Punjab, India". *Population Studies,* Vol. 44, No. 3, pp. 489-505.

Defense for Children International-USA, 1991. *The Effects of Maternal Mortality on Children in Africa: An Exploratory Report on Kenya, Namibia, Tanzania, Zambia and Zimbabwe.* DCI-USA, 1991.

Deliege, R., 1992. "Demoniac Possession among the Catholic Untouchables in Southern India". *Archives de Sciences Sociales des Religion*, Vol. 37, No. 79, pp. 115-134.

Dooley, D. 1990 (2nd ed.). *Social Research Methods.* Englewood Cliffs, New Jersey, Prentice Hall.

Douglas, M., 1966. *Purity and Danger: An Analysis of the Concepts of Pollution and Taboo*. London, Ark Paperbacks.

Dyson, T. and Moore, M., 1983. "On Kinship Structure, Female Autonomy, and

Demographic Behaviour in India". *Population and Development Review*, Vol. 9, No. 1, pp. 35-60.

Dyson, T., and Crook, N., (eds.), 1984. *India's Demography: Essays on the Contemporary Population.* New Delhi, South Asia Publishers. pp. 1-10.

Farah, A. and Preston, S., 1982. "Child Mortality Differentials in Sudan". *Population and Development Review*, Vol. 8, No. 2, pp. 365-383.

Fathalla, M. F., 1987. "The Long Road to Maternal Death". *People,* Vol. 14, No. 3, pp. 8-9.

Fathalla, M. F., Rosenfield, A., Indriso, C., Sen, D. K., and Ratnam, S. S. (eds.), 1989. *Reproductive Health: Global Issues.* Park Ridge, NJ, The Parthenon Publishing Group.

Feijoo, M. C., and Jelin E., 1989. *Women From Low Income Sectors: Economic Recession and Democratization of Politics in Argentina.* Invisible Adjustment. Santiago, UNICEF.

Flegg, A. T., 1982. "Inequality of Income, Illiteracy and Medical Care As Determinants of Infant Mortality in Underdeveloped Countries". *Population Studies,* Vol. 36, No. 3, pp. 441-58.

Flegg, A. T., 1983. "On the Determinants of Infant Mortality in Underdeveloped Countries". *International Journal of Social Economics*, Vol. 10, No. 5, pp. 38-51.

Fortney, J. A., 1987. "The Importance of Family Planning in Reducing Maternal Mortality". *Studies in Family Planning,* Vol. 18, March/April, pp. 109-114.

Frankel, S., 1980. " 'I am Dying of Man': The Pathology of Pollution". *Culture, Medicine and Psychiatry*, Vol. 4, No. 2, pp. 95-117.

Freed, R. S., and Freed, S., A., 1989. "Beliefs and Practices Resulting in Female Deaths and Fewer Females than Males in India". *Population and Environment,* Vol. 10, No. 3, pp. 144-161.

Gittelsohn, J., Bentley, M. E., Pelto, P. J., Nag, M., Pachauri, S., Harrison, A. D., and Landman, L. T., (eds.), 1994. *Listening to Women Talk about their Health: Issues and Evidence from India.* The Ford Foundation, New Delhi, Har-Anand Publications.

Gomes da-Silva, J. C., and Douglas, M., 1984. "Dual Patterns of Pollution". *Homme,* Vol. 24, No. 3-4, pp. 114-127.

Gopalan, C., 1985. "The Mother and Child in India". *Economic and Political Weekly,* Vol. 20, No. 4, pp. 162.

Government of India, 1985. *Seventh Five-Year Plan*, Planning Commission, New Delhi.

Government of India, 1987. *Health Information of India.* Central Bureau of Health Intelligence, New Delhi, Ministry of Health and Family Welfare.

Government of India, 1989. *Annual Report: 1988-89.* New Delhi, Ministry of Health and Family Welfare.

Government of India, 1994. *Economic Survey 1993-94.* New Delhi, Ministry of Finance, Economic Division.

Government of India, 1981. *Report of the Working Group on: "Health For All By*

2000 A. D.", New Delhi, Ministry of Health and Family Welfare.

Grant, J. P., 1985. *The State of the World's Children 1985.* New York, Oxford University Press.

Halstead, S. B., Walsh, J. A., and Warren, K. S. (eds.), 1985. *Good Health at Low Cost.* New York, The Rockefeller Foundation.

Healey, J. F., 1996 (4th ed). *Statistics: A Tool For Social Research.* Belmont, California, Wadsworth Publishing Company.

Hill, K., and Pebley, A. R., 1989. "Child Mortality in the Developing World". *Population and Development Review*, Vol. 15, No. 4, pp. 657-687.

Hobcraft, J. N., 1985. "World Fertility Survey: A Final Assessment". *People*, Vol. 12, pp. 3-5.

Hobcraft, J., McDonald, J. W., and Rutstein, S. O., 1984. "Socio-economic Factors in Infant and Child Mortality: A Cross-National Comparison". *Population Studies*, Vol. 38, No. 2, pp. 193-223.

Hobcraft, J., McDonald, J. W., and Rutstein, S. O., 1983. "Child-Spacing Effects on Infant and Early Child Mortality". *Population Index*, Vol. 49, No. 4, pp. 585-618.

Hobcraft, J., McDonald, J. W., and Rutstein, S. O., 1985. "Demographic Determinants of Infant and Early Child Mortality: A Comparative Analysis". *Population Studies*, Vol. 39, pp. 363- 385.

Howard, D., 1987. "Aspects of Maternal Morbidity: The Experience of Less Developed Countries". *Advances in International Maternal and Child Health*, Jelliffe, D., and Jelliffe, P. (eds.), Oxford, Clarendon Press.

Indian Council of Medical Research/Ford Foundation, 1984. *Workshop on Child Health, Nutrition and Family Planning.* Papers Presented at the Workshop held at Gauhati (September 22-24, 1983). New Delhi, Indian Council of Medical Research.

International Institute for Population Sciences (IIPS), 1995. *National Family Health Survey (MCH and Family Planning), India 1992-93.* Bombay, IIPS.

International Labour Organisation, 1980. *Report to the Copenhagen Mid-Decade Conference on Women*, Geneva, ILO.

Jain, A. K., 1985. "Determinants of Regional Variations in Infant Mortality in Rural India". *Population Studies*, Vol. 39, No. 3, pp. 407-424.

Jain, A. K., and Visaria P., 1988 (eds.). *Infant Mortality in India, Differentials and Determinants*, New Delhi, Sage Publications.

Jeffery, P., Jeffery, R., and Lyon, A., 1989. *Labour Pains and Labour Power: Women and Childbearing in India.* London, Zed Books.

Jejeebhoy, S. J., and Kulkarni, S., 1989. "Reproductive Motivation: A Comparison of Wives and Husbands in Maharashtra, India". *Studies in Family Planning*, Vol. 20, No. 5, pp. 264-272.

Joshi, N., 1979. *Cultural Factors in Health: Studies in the Sociology of Medicine in an Indian Town.* Ph.D. Thesis, Sagar University, Madhya Pradesh, India.

Kandrack M. A. *et al.*, 1991. "Gender Differences in Health Related Behaviour". *Social Science and Medicine*, Vol. 32, pp. 579-590.

Kanitkar, T., and Sinha, R. K., 1985. *Factors Associated With Increased Age At*

Marriage in Orissa. New Delhi, Population Research Centre.

Kannan, K. P., Thankappan, K. R., Raman Kutty, V., and Aravindan, K. P., 1991. *Health and Development in Rural Kerala: A Study of the Linkages Between Socioeconomic Status and Health Status*. Kerala, Kerala Sastra Sahitya Parishad.

Karkal, M., 1982. "Health For All: A Review and Critique of Two Reports". *Economic and Political Weekly*, Vol. 17, pp. 249-253.

Karkal, M., 1985. "Health of Mother and Child Survival". *Dynamics of Population and Family Welfare*, K. Srinivasan and S. Mukherji (eds.), Bombay, Himalaya Publishing House, pp. 358-374.

Karkal, M., 1987. "Differentials in Mortality by Sex". *Economic and Political Weekly*, August 8, pp. 1343-1347.

Key, P., 1987. "Women, Health and Development, With Special Reference to Indian Women". *Health Policy and Planning*, Vol. 2, No. 1, pp. 58-69.

Khan, A. R., Jahan, F. A., and Begum, S. F., 1986. "Maternal Mortality in Rural Bangladesh: The Jamalpur Distric". *Studies in Family Planning*, Vol. 17, pp. 7-12.

Khan, M. E., 1988. "Infant Mortality in Uttar Pradesh: A Micro - Level Study". *Infant Mortality in India, and Determinants*, Jain, A. K., and Visaria, P. (eds.), New Delhi, Sage Publications.

Khan, M. E., *et al.*, 1987. *Inequalities Between Men and Women in Nutrition and Family Welfare Services: An In-depth Inquiry in an Indian Village*. Population and Labour Policies Program Working Paper Number 158 (Geneva: ILO).

Khan, M. E., Ghosh Dastidar, S. K., Singh, R., 1986. "Nutrition and Health Practices Among Rural Women - A Case Study of Uttar Pradesh, India". *The Journal of Family Welfare*, Vol. 33, No. 1.

Kielmann, A. A., *et al.*, 1983. "Analysis of Morbidity and Mortality". *Child and Maternal Health Services in Rural India: The Narangwal Experiment*, A. A. Kielmann, *et al.* (eds.), Vol. 1, Baltimore, The Johns Hopkins University Press.

Kielmann, A. A., *et al.*, 1983. *Child and Maternal Health Services in Rural India: The Narangwal Experiment*. Baltimore and London, The Johns Hopkins University Press.

Kramer, E., 1987. "The Relativity of Norms". *Osterreichische Zeitschrift fur Soziologie*, Vol. 12, No. 1, pp. 93-99.

Kunitz, S. J., 1987. "Explanations and Ideologies of Mortality Patterns". *Population and Development Review*, Vol. 13, No. 3, pp. 379-408.

Lawrence, D. L., 1982. "Reconsidering the Menstrual Taboo: A Portuguese Case". *Anthropological Quarterly*, Vol. 55, No. 2, pp. 84-98.

Lee, P. L. Rance, 1978. "Interaction Between Chinese and Western Medicine in Hong Kong: Modernisation and Professional Inequality". *Culture and Healing in Asian Societies: Anthropological, Psychiatric and Public Health Studies*, A. Kleinman, P. Kunstadter, E. Russel Alexander, J. L. Gale (eds.), Cambridge, Massachusetts, Schenkman Publishing Co.

Leonard, W. L. II, 1976. *Basic Social Statistics*. St. Paul, West Publishing Company.

Loether, H. J., and McTanish, D. G., 1993 (4th ed). *Descriptive and Inferential*

Statistics. Boston, Allyn and Bacon.

Luzzi, G. E. F., 1974. "Food Avoidances during the Puerperium and Lactation in Tamil Nadu". *Economy of Food and Nutrition*, Vol. 3.

MacCormack, C. P., 1988. "Health and the Social Power of Women". *Social Science and Medicine*, Vol. 26, pp. 677-683.

Madan, T. N., 1985. "Concerning the Categories Subha and Suddha in Hindu Culture: An Exploratory Essay". *Journal of Developing Societies*, Vol. 1, No. 1, pp. 11-29.

Madan, T. N., 1987. "Community Involvement in Health Policy, Sociocultural and Dynamic Aspects of Health Beliefs". *Social Science and Medicine*, Vol. 25, No. 6, pp. 615-620.

Mahadevan, K., Reddy, P. R., Murthy, M. S. R., Reddy, P. J., Gowri, V., and Raju, S. S., 1986. "Culture, Nutrition and Mortality in South Central India". *Journal of Family Welfare*, Vol. 32, No. 3, pp. 36-58.

Mahajan, B. K., 1972, *Preventive and Social Medicine in India*, New Delhi, Jaypee Brothers.

Maine, D. *et al.*, 1987. *Prevention of Maternal Deaths in Developing Countries: Program Options and Practical Considerations*. Paper Prepared for the International Safe Motherhood Conference, Nairobi, 10-13 February.

McCarthy, J. and Maine, D., 1992. "A Framework for Analysing the Determinants of Maternal Mortality". *Studies in Family Planning*, Vol. 23, No. 1, pp. 23-33.

Miller, B. D., 1981. *The Endangered Sex: Neglect of Female Children in Rural North India*. Ithaca and London, Cornell University Press.

Mines, D. P., 1989. "Hindu Periods of Death 'Impurity'". *Contributions to Indian Sociology*, — New Series, Vol. 23, No. 1, pp. 103-130.

Ministry of Health and Family Welfare (MOHFW), 1992. *Module for Health Workers*. National Child Survival and Safe Motherhood Programme, New Delhi, MOHFW.

Misra, B. D., 1984. "Reasons for Under-Utilisation of Health Services—A Review". ICMR/Ford Foundation Workshop on Child Health, Nutrition and Family Welfare, Indian Council of Medical Research, New Delhi.

Momsen, J., 1987. "Introduction". *Geography of Gender in the Third World*, Momsen, J. and Townsend, J. (eds.), New York, State University of New York Press.

Morley, D., Rhode, J., and Williams, G., 1987, (eds.). *Practicing Health for All*. Oxford, New York, Toronto, Oxford Medical Publications, Oxford University Press.

Mosley, W. H., and Chen, L. C., 1984. "An Analytical Framework for the Study of Child Survival in Developing Countries". *Child Survival: Strategies for Research*, Mosley, W. H. and Chen, L. C. (eds.), *Population and Development Review* (Supplement to Volume 10), pp. 25-45.

Mosley, W. H., 1985. "Will Primary Health Care Reduce Infant and Child Mortality?, A Critique of Some Current Strategies, With Special Reference to Africa and Asia". *Health Policy, Social Policy and Mortality Prospects*, Vallin, J., and Lopez, A. D. (eds.), Ordina Editions, Liege. pp. 189-208.

Mudiraj, G. N. R., 1973. "Spatial Differentiation of Castes: Analysis of a Regional Pattern". *Man in India*, Vol. 53, No. 1, pp. 13-18.

Mukhopadhyay, M., 1987. "Human Development through Primary Health Care: Case Studies from India". *Practicing Health for All*, David Morley, Jon Rohde and Glen Williams (eds.), Oxford Medical Publications, Oxford University Press.

Nag, M., 1989. "Political Awareness as a Factor in Accessibility of Health Services: A Case Study of Rural Kerala and West Bengal". *Economic and Political Weekly*, Vol. 24, 1989.

Nag, M., 1983. "The Impact of Social and Economic Development on Mortality: A Comparative Study of Kerala and West Bengal". *Economic and Political Weekly*, Vol. 18, No. 19/20/21 Annual Number, pp. 877-900.

Nations, M. K., 1985. "Consideration of Cultural Factors In Child Health". *Good Health at Low Cost*, Halstead, S. B., Walsh, J. A., and Warren, K. S. (eds.), New York, The Rockefeller Foundation.

Ojanuga, D. N., and Gilbert, C., 1992. "Women's Access To Health Care in Developing Countries". *Social Science and Medicine,* Vol. 35, No. 4, pp. 613-617.

Ojanuga, D., 1991. "Preventing Birth Injury in Africa: Case Studies in Northern Nigeria". *American Journal of Orthopsychiatry,* Vol. 61, pp. 533-539.

Okojie, Christiana E. E., 1994. "Gender Inequalities of Health in the Third World". *Social Science and Medicine*, Vol. 39, No. 9, pp. 1237-1247.

Padmanabha, P., 1982. "Mortality in India: A Note on Trends and Implications". *Economic and Political Weekly,* Vol. 17, No. 32, pp. 1285-1290.

Paige, K. E., and Paige, J. M., 1981. *The Politics of Reproductive Ritual.* Berkeley, University of California Press.

Park, J. E., and Park, K., 1991, *Textbook of Preventive and Social Medicine*, Banaraidas Bhanot Publishers, Jabalpur, India.

Pebley, A. R., 1984. "Intervention Projects and the Study of Socioeconomic Determinants of Mortality". *Population and Development Review,* Vol. 10, Supplement, pp. 281-305.

Pelto, G. H., 1987. "Cultural Issues in Maternal and Child Health and Nutrition". *Social Science and Medicine,* Vol. 25, No. 6, pp. 553-559.

Perera, T., 1983. "Perinatal Morbidity and Mortality Trends in South East Asia". Proceedings of the *ASEAN Pediatric Federation Workshop on Perinatal Morbidity and Mortality*, Kuala Lumpur, 6-7 June. In *ASEAN Perinatal Health Issues*. H. Abdul Kadir (ed.), Kuala Lumpur, ASEAN Pediatric Federation.

Pool, R., 1984. *Avoidances and the Hot/Cold Syndrome: Case Study in Rural Gujarat, India.* ZZOA Working Paper No. 39, Universiteit Van Amsterdam, Dept. of South and South East Asian Studies, Anthropology and Sociology Centre. University of Amsterdam.

Potter, J. E., 1988. "Birth Spacing and Child Survival: A Cautionary Note Regarding the Evidence From the World Fertility Survey". *Population Studies,* Vol. 42, pp. 443-450.

Puentes-Markides, C., 1992. "Women and Access to Health Care". *Social Science and Medicine,* Vol. 35, No. 4, pp. 619-626.

Puffer, R. R., and Griffin, G. W., 1967. *Patterns of Urban Mortality*. Washington,

DC, Pan American Health Organisation.

Puffer, R. R., Rice, R., and Serrano, C. V., 1973. *Patterns of Mortality In Childhood*, Scientific Publication No. 262, Washington, Pan American Health Organisation.

Rao, B. K., 1985. "Maternal Mortality in India: A Review". Paper Presented at the Inter-Regional Meeting on the Prevention of Maternal Mortality, Geneva, 11-15 November, World Health Organization Document No. FHE/PMM/85.9.4.

Rao, B. K., and Malika, P. E., 1977. "A Study of Maternal Mortality in Madras City". *Journal of Obstetrics and Gynaecology of India,* Vol. 27, No. 6, pp. 876-880.

Rao, P. S. S., and Richard J., 1984. "Socioeconomic and Demographic Correlates of Medical Care and Health Practices". *Journal of Biosocial Science,* Vol. 16, No. 3, pp. 343-355.

Rao, S., 1979. "Attitudes to Women and Nutrition Programs in India". *Lancet,* Vol. 2, pp. 1357.

Ravindran S., 1986. *Health Implications of Sex Discrimination In Childhood.* World Health Organisation/UNICEF Document, WHO/UNICEF/FHE86.2.

Registrar-General, 1988. *Sample Registration Bulletin No. 22*, Vital Statistics Division, Office of the Registrar-General, New Delhi, India.

Registrar-General, 1988. *Sample Registration System, 1986*, Vital Statistics Division, Office of the Registrar-General, New Delhi, India.

Rochat, R. W., 1981. "Maternal Mortality in the United States of America". *World Health Statistics Quarterly,* Vol. 34, No. 1, pp. 2-13.

Rosen, L. N., 1973. "Contagion and Cataclysm: A Theoretical Approach to the Study of Ritual Pollution Beliefs". *African Studies,* Vol. 32, No. 4, pp. 229-246.

Roy, S., 1986. *Technical Paper 4: Development and Use of Indicators and Information Relating to Maternal and Child Health Care in India*, National Institute of Health and Family Welfare, New Delhi.

Royston, E., and Armstrong, S., 1989 (eds.). *Preventing Maternal Deaths.* Geneva, World Health Organisation.

Rutstein, S. O., 1984. *Infant and Child Mortality: Levels, Trends and Demographic Differentials. Comparative Studies: Cross-National Summaries*, No. 43, Revised Edition, London, World Fertility Survey.

Rutter, M., 1988. "Women and Health in Developing Countries". *Nursing,* Vol. 25, pp. 935-936.

Ruzicka, L. T., and Chowdhury, A. K. M. A., 1978. *Demographic Surveillance System in Matlab,* Vital Events and Migration 1974 (Section C), Cholera Research Laboratory Science, Report No. 11, Dhaka.

Sadik, N., 1989. *Investing in Women: The Focus of the '90s.* New York, United Nations Population Fund (UNFPA).

Schultz, T. P., 1989. "Investments in Women, Economic Development and Improvements In Health In Low Income Countries". *Annals NY Academy of Science,* Vol. 569, pp. 288-310.

Semi, E. T., 1985. "The Beta Israel (Falashas): From Purity to Impurity". *Jewish Journal of Sociology,* Vol 27, No. 2, pp. 103-114.

Sen, A., and Sengupta, S., 1983. "Malnutrition of Rural Children and the Sex Bias". *Economic and Political Weekly,* Vol. 18, 1983.

Seymour-Smith, C., 1986. *MacMillan Dictionary of Anthropology.* London, The MacMillan Press Ltd.

Shariff, Abusaleh., 1987. "Child Survival: A Village-Level Investigation of Some Cultural Factors Associated with Morbidity and Mortality in South India". *Human Organisation,* Vol. 46, No. 4, pp. 348-355.

Simmons, G. B., Smucker, C. M., Misra, B. D., and Majumdar, P., 1978. "Patterns and Causes of Infant Mortality In Rural Uttar Pradesh". *Journal of Tropical Paediatrics and Environment Child Health,* Vol. 27, No. 5, pp. 207.

Sinha, U. P., 1990. "Child Mortality in India: Some Facts and Issues". *Dynamics of Population and Family Welfare,* K. Srinivasan and K. B. Pathak (eds.), Bombay, Himalaya Publishing House.

Sivard R., 1985. *Women's Health. Women: A World Survey,* World Priorities, Washington, DC, 1985.

Smyke, P., 1991. *Women and Health.* London and New Jersey, Zed Books.

Sopher, D. E.,1980 (ed.). *An Exploration of India: Geographical Perspectives on Society and Culture.* London, Longman Group.

Srinivasan, K., and Mukherji, S., 1985. "Health of Mother and Child Survival". *Dynamics of Population and Family Welfare,* K. Srinivasan and K. B. Pathak (eds.), Bombay, Himalaya Publishing House, pp. 358-374.

Stinson, W., 1986. *Women and Health.* World Federation of Public Health, 1986.

Stock, R., 1983. "Distance and the Utilisation of Health Care Facilities in Rural Nigeria". *Social Science and Medicine,* Vol. 17, pp. 563-570.

Subedi, J., 1989. "Modern Health Services and Health Care Behaviour: A Survey in Kathmandu, Nepal". *Journal of Health and Social Behaviour,* Vol. 30, pp. 412-420.

Sundari, T. K., 1992, "The Untold Story: How The Health Care Systems in Developing Countries Contribute to Maternal Mortality". *International Journal of Health Services,* Vol. 22, No. 3, pp. 513-528.

Thaddeus, S. and Maine, D., 1990. *Too Far to Walk: Maternal Mortality in Context.* New York, Columbia University, Centre for Population and Family Health.

Thompson, C., 1985. "The Power to Pollute and the Power to Preserve: Perceptions of Female Power in a Hindu Village". *Social Science and Medicine,* Vol. 21, No. 6, pp. 701-711.

Trussell, J., and Pebley, A. R., 1984. "The Potential Impact of Changes in Fertility on Infant, Child, and Maternal Mortality". *Studies in Family Planning,* Vol. 15, No. 6, pp. 267-280.

Tuladhar, J., 1987. "Effect of Family Planning Availability and Accessibility on Contraceptive Use in Nepal". *Studies in Family Planning,* Vol. 18, pp. 49-53.

Ullrich, H. E., 1992. "Menstrual Taboos Among Havik Brahmin Women: A Study of Ritual Change". *Sex Roles,* Vol. 26, No. 1-2, pp. 19-40.

UNICEF, 1984. *An Analysis of the Situation of Children in India,* New Delhi.

UNICEF, 1986. *The State of the World's Children*. Oxford, UK, Oxford University Press.

United Nations Department of International Economic and Social Affairs, 1983. "Update: Mortality and Health Policy". *Population Division of the United Nations Population Fund*, Vol. 10, No. 3, pp. 6-30.

United Nations Fund for Population Studies (UNFPA), 1988. *UNFPA 1988 Report*. New York.

United Nations Population Fund (UNFPA), 1990. "Safe Motherhood Conference", Lahore, Pakistan, March, 1990. *Population, UNFPA Newsletter*, Vol. 16, No. 5, pp. 3.

United Nations Secretariat, 1984. "Mortality and Health Policy: Main Issues for the 1980s". *Population Bulletin of the United Nations* (UN), No. 16, pp. 40-61.

United Nations, 1986. *Report of the Working Group on Traditional Practices Affecting the Health of Women and Children*. Commission on Human Rights, Doc. E/CN.4/1986/42, Processed.

Vallin, J., and Lopez, A. D., 1985, (eds.). *Health Policy, Social Policy and Mortality Prospects*, International Union for the Scientific Study of Population (IUSSP).

Visaria L., 1985. "Infant Mortality in India: Levels, Trends and Determinants". *Economic and Political Weekly*, Vol. 20, No. 32.

Vlassoff, C., 1988. "The Value of Sons in an Indian Village: How Widows See it". Paper Presented at Meeting of the Canadian Population Society, Windsor, Ontario, Canada.

Vlassoff, C., 1994. "Gender Inequalities in Health in the Third World: Uncharted Ground". *Social Science and Medicine*, Vol. 39, No. 9, pp. 1249-1259.

Ware, H., 1984. "Effects of Maternal Education, Women's Roles, and Child Care on Child Mortality". *An Analytical Framework for the Study of Child Survival in Developing Countries, Child Survival: Strategies for Research*, W. H. Mosley and L. C. Chen (eds.), *Supplement to Population and Development Review*, Vol. 10, pp. 25-45.

Winikoff, B., 1983. "The Effects of Birth Spacing on Child and Maternal Health". *Studies in Family Planning*, Vol. 14, No. 10, pp. 231-245.

Winikoff, B., 1988, "Women's Health: An Alternative Perspective For Choosing Interventions". *Studies in Family Planning*, Vol. 19, No. 4, pp. 197-214.

Winikoff, B., and Sullivan, M., 1987. "Assessing the Role of Family Planning in Reducing Maternal Mortality". *Studies in Family Planning*, Vol. 18, No. 3, pp. 128-143.

Wolfe, B. L., and Behrman, J. R., 1984. "Determinants of Women's Health Status and Health Care Utilisation in a Developing Country: A Latent Variable Approach". *The Review of Economics and Statistics*, Vol. 66, No. 4, pp. 696-703.

Woortmann, K., 1986. "Food, Family and the Construction of the Feminine Gender". *Dados*, Vol. 29, No. 1, pp. 103-130.

World Bank, 1980. *World Development Report*. Washington, DC, The World Bank.

World Health Organisation Secretariat, 1976. "Community Water Supply and Excreta

Disposal in Developing Countries: Review of Progress". *World Health Statistics Report*, Vol. 29, No. 10, pp. 544-603

World Health Organisation, 1977. *International Classification of Diseases. Manual of International Statistical Classification of Diseases, Injuries and Causes of Death.* Geneva, WHO.

World Health Organisation, 1985. *Prevention of Maternal Mortality.* Report of A WHO Inter-Regional Meeting, Geneva, WHO.

World Health Organisation, 1985a. "Review and Appraisal: Health". Paper Presented at the United Nations Conference on Women's Decade, Nairobi. A/Conf; 116/5.

World Health Organisation, 1985b. "The United Nations Decade for Women: An End and A Beginning". *WHO Chronicle*, Vol. 35, pp. 163-170.

World Health Organisation, 1985c. *Women, Health and Development* (A Report by the Director-General). Geneva, WHO Offset Publication No. 90, 1985.

World Health Organisation, 1986a. *Maternal Mortality Rates: A Tabulation of Available Information.* Geneva, WHO.

World Health Organisation, 1986b. *Bulletin of Regional Health Information.* Delhi, WHO/Southeast Asia Regional Office.

World Health Organisation, 1992. *Women, Health and Development In the South-East Asia Region*, Regional Health Paper, SEARO, No. 22, New Delhi, pp. 22.

Wouters, A. V., 1992. "Health Care Utilisation Patterns in Developing Countries: Role of the Technology environment in "Deriving" the Demand for Health Care". *Bulletin of the World Health Organisation (WHO)*, Vol. 70, No. 3, pp. 381-389.

Appendix

Basic Indicators for India

Basic Indicators, 1990

Under 5 mortality Rate (U5MR)	142
Infant Mortality Rate (IMR)	94
Total Population (in millions)	853.1
Annual Number of Births (thousands)	26985
Annual Number of Under 5 Deaths (thousands)	3835
GNP Per Capita (US$) 1989	340
Life Expectancy at Birth (Years)	59
Total Adult Literacy Rate	48
Percentage of Age Group enrolled in Primary School (Total) 1986-1989	99

Nutrition Indicators, 1990

Percentage of infants with Low Birth Weight (LBW)	30
Percentage of Children Suffering from: (a) Underweight (0-4 Years)	
(i) Moderate and Severe	61x
(ii) Severe	9x

Health Indicators, 1990

Percentage of Population with Access to Safe Water (1988-1990)

Total	75
Rural	73
Urban	79

Percentage fully Immunised 1981/1989-90 (One Year Old Children)

TB	12/97
DPT	31/92
Polio	93
Measles	../87
Pregnant Women Tetanus	24/77
Oral Rehydration Therapy (ORT) Use Rate (1987-1989)	13

Education Indicators, 1990

Adult Literacy Rate (1990)

Male	62
Female	34

Number of Sets per 1000 Population, 1988

Radio	78
Television	7x

Primary School Enrollment Ratio 1986-1989 (Gross)

Male	114
Female	83

Primary School Enrollment Ratio 1986-1989 (Net)

Male	..
Female	..

Percentage of Grade 1 Enrollment reaching Final Grade of Primary School 1985-87   40*

Secondary School Enrollment Ratio 1986-89 (Gross)

Male	50

Female   29

Demographic Indicators, 1990

Population (millions), Under 5	114.4
Population Annual Growth Rate (%) 1989-90	2.1
Crude Death Rate (CDR)	11
Crude Birth Rate (CBR)	32
Life Expectancy (e)	59
Total Fertility Rate (TFR)	4.2
Percentage Population Urbanised (1990)	27
Average Annual Growth Rate of Urban Population (%), 1980-1990	3.7

Economic Indicators, 1990

GNP Per Capita (US$) 1989	340
GNP Per Capita Average Annual	
Growth Rate (Percentage), 1980-1989	3.2
Rate of Inflation (Percentage), 1980-1989	8
Percentage of Population Below Absolute Poverty Level, 1980-1989	
Urban	29*
Rural	33*
Percentage of Central Government Expenditure Allocated to (1986-1990)Health	2
Education	3
Defense	19

Women Indicators, 1990

Life Expectancy of Females as a Percentage of Males	100.0
Adult Literacy Rate of Females as a Percentage of Males	55
Enrollment Ratios of Females as a Percentage of Males	
Primary School	73
Secondary School	58
Contraceptive Prevalence (Percentage), 1980-1990	34
Pregnant Women Immunized Against Tetanus (1989-1990)	77
Percentage of Births Attended by Trained Health Personnel (1983-1990)	33
Maternal Mortality Rate (MMR), 1980-1990	460

Source: Sample Registration System: Fertility and Mortality Indicators, 1991; State of the World's Children, UNICEF, 1992; and Family Welfare Yearbook, 1989-1990.